ARTHRITIS & RHEUMATISM

A SELF-HELP GUIDE

COMBINING ORTHODOX AND COMPLEMENTARY APPROACHES TO HEALTH

ARTHRITIS & RHEUMATISM

A SELF-HELP GUIDE
COMBINING ORTHODOX AND COMPLEMENTARY APPROACHES TO HEALTH

HASNAIN WALJI & DR ANDREA KINGSTON

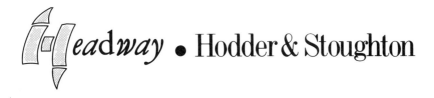

Headway • Hodder & Stoughton

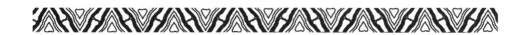

Cataloguing in Publication Data is available from the British Library

ISBN 0 340 60563 4

First published 1994
Impression number 10 9 8 7 6 5 4 3 2 1
Year   1998 1997 1996 1995 1994

Printed in Great Britain for Hodder & Stoughton Educational, a division of Hodder Headline Plc, 338 Euston Road, London NW1 3BH by Page Bros (Norwich) Ltd.

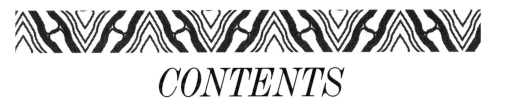

CONTENTS

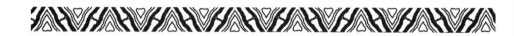

*This book is dedicated to the seekers of health
and to those who help them find it.*

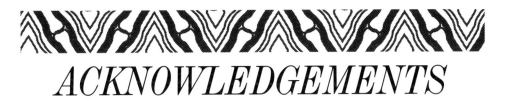

ACKNOWLEDGEMENTS

I should like to express my gratitude to Dr Andrea Kingston for her valuable input and the enlightened way she dealt with a number of apparent contradictions between orthodox medicine and complementary therapies; to nutritionist Angela Dowden for offering many pertinent suggestions; to Sato Liu of the Natural Medicines Society for her assistance in providing contacts and arranging interviews with practitioners; and to my agent Susan Mears for her encouragement and practical help.

This book could not possibly have been written without the co-operation of the following practitioners who have so willingly endured my interruptions: aromatherapy – Christine Wildwood; naturopathy – Jan De Vries; homoeopathy – Michael Thompson and Beth MacEoin; reflexology – Pauline Wills; and anthroposophical medicine – Dr Maurice Orange.

I must thank my daughter Sukaina for giving her time during vacation from university for wading through research papers and books and extracting relevant information. Last but not least, I wish to thank my wife Latifa whose gentle care and concern, not to mention long hours typing the manuscript, enabled me to complete this book.

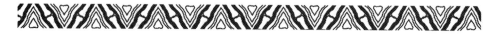

Foreword To The Series
from the Natural Medicines Society

When we visit our doctor's surgery and are given a diagnosis, we often receive a prescription at the same time. More people than ever are now aware that there may be complementary treatments available and would like to explore the possibilities, but do not know which kind of treatment would be most useful for their problem.

There are books on just about every treatment available, but few which start from this standpoint: the patient interested in knowing the options for treating their particular condition – which treatment is available or useful, what the treatment involves, or what to expect when consulting the practitioner.

The Headway Healthwise series will provide the answers for those wishing to consider what treatment is available, once the doctor has diagnosed their condition. Each book will cover both the orthodox and complementary approaches. Although patients are naturally most interested in relieving their immediate symptoms, the books show how complementary treatment goes much deeper; underlying causes are explored and the patient is treated as a whole.

It is important to stress that it is not the intention of this series to replace the expertise of the doctors and practitioners, nor to encourage self-treatment, but to show the options available to the patient.

As the consumer charity working for freedom of choice in medicine, the Natural Medicines Society welcomes the Headway Healthwise series. Although the Natural Medicines Society does not recommend people who are taking prescribed orthodox medicines to stop doing so, our aim is to introduce them to complementary forms of treatment. We believe the orthodox system of medicine is often best used as a last, not first, resort when other, gentler, methods fail or are inappropriate.

Giving patients the information to make their choice is the purpose of this series. With the increasing use of complementary medicine within the NHS, knowing the complementary options is vital both to the patients and to their doctors in the search for better health care.

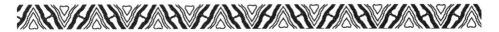

Foreword To The Book

Arthritis and rheumatism are the most common and widespread diseases to which human flesh is heir. And it is appropriate to use the word 'heir', because the main reason why these conditions are so very common is evolution. Our species, *Homo sapiens*, has evolved with dramatic speed over the last couple of million years. One of the most important evolutionary changes has been the bipedal, or upright, two-legged gait. This was an important advance because it freed our hands which, in conjunction with our massive brains, have been responsible for most of the accomplishments (as well as disasters!) for which mankind has been responsible.

But a couple of million years is a very short time in evolutionary terms, and parts of our bodies, especially our skeletons, have simply not caught up. This is the basic reason why arthritis of weight-bearing joints is so common. This applies particularly to our backs, but also to other weight-bearing joints such as hips, knees and feet. And of course, large brains are heavy, and our necks have to carry them.

This is not the whole story; other serious and common rheumatic diseases, such as rheumatoid arthritis, are more puzzling. Its cause is unknown, but its frequency is remarkably constant – it affects about 1 per cent of people all over the world. Some experts think rheumatoid arthritis is a fairly new disease, perhaps originating in the seventeenth century, making it a so-called 'disease of civilisation'.

It is certainly true that the impact of arthritic and rheumatic disease on people's lives is increasing. This is partly a case of medicine becoming a victim of its own success. Most of the diseases come on in middle or later life and are progressive, so that they affect older people more than younger. Because of social improvements and medical advances, more and more people are living to a ripe old age and the problems associated with arthritis and rheumatism are growing.

Medicine is also becoming a victim of its own success in other, understandably less well-publicised, ways. The pharmaceutical industry recently passed a minor landmark with the introduction of the first 'designer chaser drug' – the first drug designed purely to counteract the side-effects of another drug. The drug counteracts the stomach irritation frequently caused by non-steroidal

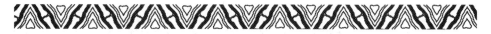

anti-inflammatory drugs (NSAIDs), the most commonly used group of drugs for arthritic and rheumatic complaints.

Meanwhile the benefits of complementary therapies are increasingly recognised by doctors, scientists and government. About 300,000 patients per year are referred to hospital for treatment of back pain every year; a recent research project showed that the use of chiropractic for such patients might save 290,000 days off sick, and this would save £2.9 m in social security payments and £13 m in lost output. Osteopaths have recently been recognised by the government as a registered health profession and chiropractors will probably soon follow suit.

In the midst of all this change it is difficult to find sensible, balanced advice on the nature of the illnesses, the pros and cons of the various possible conventional and complementary treatments, and how to go about getting them. *Arthritis and Rheumatism* starts by describing how healthy joints work, and explains in easily understood terms the nature of the main rheumatic diseases. It goes on to give a balanced account of what you should and should not expect from conventional treatment. The rest of the book is a thorough explanation of the main forms of complementary medicine and what they have to offer to people suffering from arthritis and rheumatism. This book will be useful to anybody suffering from the painful and disabling arthritic and rheumatic conditions, and I warmly recommend it.

Dr. Peter Fisher MRCP FFHom
Consultant Physician, Royal London Homoeopathic Hospital.
Lecturer in Rheumatology and Complementary Medicine,
St Bartholomew's Hospital Medical College.
Member of the Natural Medicines Society's Medicines Advisory
Research Committee.

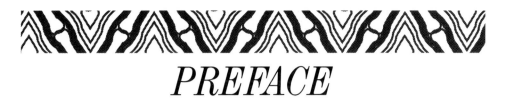

PREFACE

Headway Healthwise is a concise new series which takes the original approach of looking at common ailments and describing how they may be treated using complementary therapies. The aim of the series is not to replace the orthodox medical approach but to give readers an overview of how they may be helped by consulting complementary practitioners.

Once a condition has been diagonised by a GP, those wishing to avail themselves of other forms of treatment will find this book particularly useful. The intention of this series is not to recommend people taking prescribed orthodox medicines to stop taking these. It is to introduce them to alternative and complementary forms of treatment which may enable them reduce the amount of orthodox prescriptions, at the very least, and, in many cases, do away with their need altogether.

We have attempted to present the information in a style that is clear and easy to read. The central approach is to look at addiction from different perspectives by providing you with descriptions of several complementary therapies. While cautioning against self-medication, the book has been written to encourage you to take charge of your own health by making an informed choice of therapy. It shows how and why orthodox medicine – a life-saving and useful system of medicine – should be used as a last resort when other more natural methods fail, rather than the first recourse.

An overview of arthritis and rheumatism in the opening chapter is followed by a chapter on the kind of treatment to expect from your GP. The second chapter deals with such factors as lifestyle, diet and nutrition in the management of the disorder. Later chapters look at complementary approaches to the subject.

The one common factor that underpins all the alternative or complementary therapeutic techniques described in this book is the belief in the healing power of the body. Practitioners recognise that the body possesses an inherent ability to cure itself. This gives a clear message to the patient of his/her role in the healing process – that of the mind willing the body to heal itself.

At first sight this may appear to challenge the approach of orthodox medicine, in which the therapeutic objective is to cure the

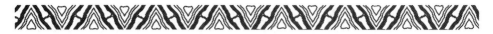

diseased part of the body. The patient has no role to play except dutifully to take the medicine. The concept of a white-coated god who possesses the magic pill to cure is the result of fear combined with a lack of understanding of the nature of disease and, more so, that of health.

This book is an attempt to dispel myths and to bring about a greater understanding of the issues relating to health and healing, which go beyond the realms of simple anatomy and biology. The recognition that orthodox medicine and complementary therapies need not be mutually exclusive, as both have a role to play, can go a long way towards promoting the integrated medicine of the twenty-first century.

Hasnain Walji
Milton Keynes
March, 1994

Note: Any information given in this book is not intended to be taken as a replacement for medical advice. Any person with a condition requiring medical attention should consult a medical professional.

Throughout the book you will find some words in italics. If these are not immediately explained, you will find the explanation in the glossary.

1
OVERVIEW: MACHINE MAINTENANCE WITH A DIFFERENCE

Proverbially, 'lifting a finger' describes the smallest of actions. Little do we realise that when we move a finger, a well-engineered part of our body performs a complicated routine. Robotics engineers tell us how difficult it is to emulate the perfect co-ordination of even the simplest of human joint movements. Our *musculoskeletal system* (the bones, muscles and joints in our bodies) enable us to move about – something we very much take for granted.

For any mechanical device, reliability and long, trouble-free service depends upon good design complemented by well-made and durable components. However, even the best-designed machine with the most rugged components will not last long without careful, appropriate use and a maintenance programme. This also applies to the human body – but a maintenance programme for the musculoskeletal system has to take into account the mind and spirit in addition to physical maintenance.

Fractures, torn *ligaments* (white tissue that links two bones together at a joint) and *pulled* (strained) muscles are all examples of overtaxing the musculoskeletal system. Such ailments as *tennis elbow* (inflammation of the elbow) or *housemaid's knee* (inflammation and swelling of the knee) are caused by overuse of joints.

Rheumatism is a general term for pain emanating from the joints or structures around them while *arthritis*, which literally means 'inflammation', is commonly used for any type of joint disease. Although there are many different types of arthritis, the two major ones are *osteoarthritis* and *rheumatoid arthritis*.

Osteoarthritis is the most common kind, affecting one in ten of the UK population. It is caused by general wear and tear of the body. A relatively mild condition, osteoarthritis affects the knees, fingers, hips and sometimes the spine.

Rheumatoid arthritis is less common but appears to affect younger people and is associated with problems of the immune system. Rheumatoid arthritis affects the joints, muscles and even the heart and lungs in rare cases; it is more serious than osteoarthritis. In order to understand how these movement-limiting disorders are caused, let us look at the strikingly functional design and structure of our joints which allow us to move almost as soon as the mind wills – and sometimes even before, as in the case of a reflex action.

The Capsule Of Movement

Essentially, a joint is a mechanical device. Bone is a living tissue made up of a form of protein which binds calcium, magnesium and phosphorus. The shape of the bones in the joint enables a wide range of movement. Some joints are like a hinge (knee and elbow) while others are like a ball and socket (hip and shoulder).

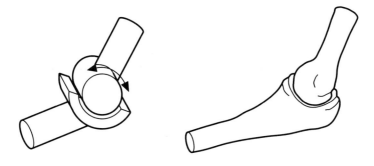

The elbow, a hinge joint

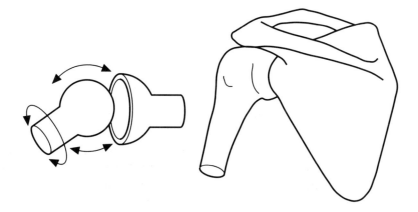

The shoulder, a ball and socket joint

Cartilage is the glistening smooth layer on the bone-ends in the joint. It is made from protein and carbohydrate. Because it is smooth and less brittle than the bone, it assists in joint movements. It also works as a shock absorber.

The joint is encompassed by a thin membrane called the *synovial membrane* which contains *synovial fluid* – lubricating liquid produced in synovial cells and secreted into the joint space to 'oil' the joints.

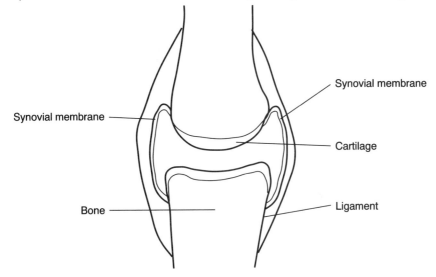

Normal joint, showing the cushion of cartilage and synovial fluid

Ligaments are strong fibres which strengthen the outer synovial membrane and contribute to the stability of the joint.

Outside this capsule there are muscles which are attached to the bones by *tendons* (sinews). Small fluid-filled sacs, called the *bursa*, help to reduce friction between the tendons and bones, particularly when they are very close to the skin.

Joint Disorders

Disorders affecting the bone, cartilage, the synovial membrane, as well as the muscles, tendons and bursa are all classified under the general heading of diseases of the joints. When the disorders are related to the surrounding tissue, such as tendons, ligaments and bursa, they are called *periarticular disorders*. Torn ligaments, a sprained ankle, housemaid's knee and tennis elbow fall into this category. Most of these conditions cause pain in a particular spot, although it may spread around the area, which gets better after a

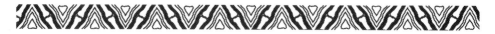

while. *Fibrositis* (also known as *muscular rheumatism*) is another type of periarticular disorder where pain comes from the muscles surrounding the joints.

On the other hand, *articular disorders* (arthritis) are those which are generally confined to disease of the joint itself. There are almost 200 different kinds of arthritis, (as many as the number of joints in the body). However, as we explained a moment ago, most of them can be classified under one or other of the following:

- damage to the surface cartilage and bone as in osteoarthritis;
- inflammation of the synovial membrane as in rheumatoid arthritis.

Osteoarthritis (OA)

This involves the breakdown in the surface of the joint, usually of the cartilage and sometimes even the bone. Affecting the joints of the hands and feet as well as the hips, this disease is caused by damage to the cartilage and, in extreme cases, even the bones, leading to excess friction and overuse. Almost 5 million people in Britain suffer from OA with symptoms commonly appearing at about the age of 50. Although it is usually a mild condition it can cause severe joint damage resulting in pain and disability and is therefore the single biggest cause of disability in this country. Some families are more prone to this disorder than others, as indeed are overweight people.

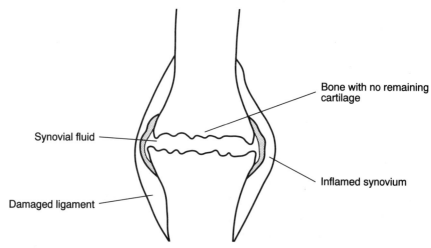

Osteoarthritic joint, showing the pitted bone and lack of cartilage

How Does It Occur?

It begins when the cartilage surface in the joint becomes roughened and the process of thinning leads to the further breakdown of the cartilage. In some case the cartilage may almost disappear from the bone ends. The shape of the bone ends begins to change when the *collagen* (the protein matrix of the bone) breaks down. Large bone spurs, called *osteophytes,* then form at the edges of the bone. The distorted appearance of the hands of sufferers is a result of these outgrowths. The synovial fluid also becomes thinner and increasingly less able to lubricate the joint. Consequently the synovial membrane and the rest of the joint becomes inflamed and movement becomes restricted.

Why Does It Occur?

There are a number of factors which contribute to OA: ageing, genetic make-up, wear and tear, bad posture (particularly where the joint is weak or the structure is abnormal). It is good to know that the extra demands made on the joints during sport and exercise do not in themselves cause OA. However, a succession of sports injuries relating to the joints can be a contributory factor to OA, for example, knee injuries in a footballer. Rheumatoid arthritis and gout can also result in OA. This is called *secondary OA.*

Rheumatoid Arthritis (RA)

This condition can be crippling in severe cases and can cause a number of complications. It is estimated that over half a million people suffer from it in this country, the majority of whom are women. RA most often affects fingers, wrists, knees and ankles.

How does it occur?

RA begins with the inflammation of the synovial membrane. The whole joint becomes becomes hot, swollen and painful because excess fluid leaks out of the inflamed membrane. As the disease progresses, a process of cartilage and bone degeneration begins, leading to permanent damage and deformity of the joints.

Like the synovial membrane, inflammation can occur in the linings of the tendons and the bursae, making movement painful and difficult. The tendons may occasionally snap or develop nodules

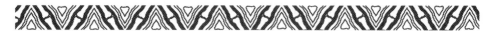

just under the skin. Not just the linings in the joints, but other parts of the body are affected, too. In RA the lining of the heart, lungs, kidneys and even the eyes can be affected.

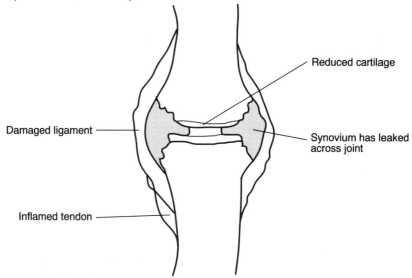

Rheumatoid arthritic joint, showing the synovium spread across the joint surface

Why Does It Occur?

Unlike OA, there are a number of mysterious factors. Environmental and genetic factors are thought to trigger RA. Several genes have been identified that predispose certain people to RA. The environmental factors are more difficult to identify, as there are many types of pollutants which could be responsible. Recent medical thinking has focused upon *autoimmune diseases* and RA is considered to be one of them. An autoimmune disease is one which the immune system, which normally protects us against infection, reacts against the body itself. This will be described later in this chapter.

Ankylosing Spondylitis (AS)

This tongue-twisting term is used for arthritis when the joints in the back become inflamed and stiffen up. *Ankylosing* means 'stiff joints' and *spondylitis* means 'inflammation of the spine'. It is a condition that usually affects young adult men, although women can be afflicted by it too.

How Does It Occur?

AS begins with inflammation of the ends of ligaments and tendons where they are attached to the bone. One difference from RA is that the inflammatory reaction turns to scar tissue, which eventually turns into bone. This bone growth bridges the gap between the *vertebrae* (the bones in the spine)so that part of the bone becomes rigid. This is what causes stiffness in the spine.

Why Does It Occur?

The cause is still a mystery for modern medical science but it is believed that environmental causes trigger the onset of the disease in those who are genetically predisposed to it.

Gout

Traditionally, a disease that has been associated with good living and too much port, it is, in fact, the result of a build up of uric acid crystals in the joints, thereby causing an inflammation. Gout does not discriminate between men and women; however, it does run in families and usually sets in during middle age.

How Does It Occur?

Gout often starts with an acute attack in the big toe. Uric acid should be excreted from the body via the kidneys. If there is excess uric acid in the blood it is deposited in the form of crystals in the joints. Uric acid crystals, growing in the cartilage, produce a small lump of chalky material. The crystals fall into the joint space and inflammation begins.

Why Does It Occur?

In addition to genetic factors, consumption of foods or drink that make uric acid in the body causes gout. Sometimes drugs or kidney damage may also raise uric acid levels in the blood.

What Is An Autoimmune Disease?

The human immune system has amazing capabilities when it comes to fighting foreign organisms which cause illness. In order to fight

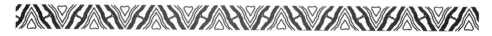

disease, it is required to distinguish between cells which are foreign and cells which are not.

As soon as the immune system encounters something that it perceives as foreign, certain cells in the body fight the organism to get rid of it. The system is so sophisticated that it can actually remember the foreign organism and is able to respond to it more quickly the next time it is encountered. This is called *acquired immunity.*

Vaccination is a good example of one way in which we can acquire immunity. A small amount of treated or dead organism is introduced into the body by injecting a vaccine. As the organism is already treated or dead, there is no danger of acquiring the disease. However, as soon as the body's defence force encounters it, it is put on red alert, fights it and makes *antibodies* (proteins which render foreign organisms harmless) to it. The immune system will also remember how to get rid of the organism should it meet a similar one in the future. So, if you were to become infected with an active live organism of the same kind, say of cholera, your immune system would be able to respond to it before the foreign organism had a chance to cause disease. All the information is stored in the *thymus gland,* the body's 'computer'. It instructs the body's defence force when to commence attack and, equally, when not to attack in the case of harmless foreign organisms.

As long as the immune system is healthy it can fend off the onslaught of disease. But it can be compromised by poor diet, environmental pollution, stress and even the natural process of ageing, with serious consequences.

Sometimes when the immune system malfunctions it becomes overactive and starts attacking harmless foreign substances. Hay fever is a classic example of an overactive immune system. Normally, pollen is harmless and yet the immune system starts to attack pollen particles. The cells involved in *allergic response* come out in full force releasing *histamine,* resulting in the symptoms of hay fever. Problems also arise in transplants because the immune system, programmed to reject a foreign tissue, begins to attack the new heart or kidney.

At times, the immune system goes horribly wrong and actually starts attacking the body's own cells. Rheumatoid arthritis is just such an example. Termed an autoimmune disease, it is among a number of autoimmune disorders such as *diabetes mellitus, multiple sclerosis* and *lupus.* It cannot distinguish between 'self' (the body's own cells) and 'non-self' (foreign organisms) and tries to produce

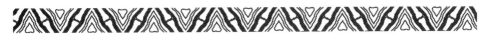

antibodies against its own cells. White blood cells are the complex organisms that form our defensive arsenal. They are divided into subgroups, each with a specific responsibility to defend us against the onslaught of disease. The *T-cells* (*T-lymphocytes*), for example, have a regulatory function. The *B-cells* (*B-lymphocytes*) secrete highly effective antibodies. If there is a breakdown in any of the components of the immune system, the body's ability to fight disease is severely impaired. The result is that many of us live with recurring health problems – colds, 'flu, chronic fatigue and other diseases, including hay fever and asthma.

Autoimmune disease occurs when the body starts to produce antibodies against its own cells. Both the T-cells and the B-cells can malfunction and the system begins to pursue its own tissue. The causes for this confusion are ageing, pollution and *free radicals.* Oxygen is necessary to sustain life but, paradoxically, is also a cause of health problems. All living things that use oxygen also produce free radicals. When cells use oxygen, they inevitably produce a small proportion of unstable molecules that lack an electron (molecules are stable only when they are electronically even). These unstable oxygen molecules are free radicals. Created every minute we are alive, they are largely held in check by the body's army of *antioxidants* (see Chapter 3) and, as long as the free radicals are kept under control, we remain healthy. However, if we begin to make more free radicals than we need (and they do serve a useful function), there is a risk of damage to the immune system and of developing chronic diseases. As well as playing a role in rheumatoid arthritis, unchecked free radicals are also thought to be a contributory cause of mutations and cancers, memory loss and senility.

Neutralising Free Radicals

Because free radicals can be hazardous to human health it is important to neutralise them before they do any damage. The defences against free radicals are antioxidants, which mop up excess free radicals by binding to them and thus neutralising their potentially damaging effects. Commonly recognised antioxidants are vitamins C and E, and the pro-vitamin A, beta carotene and the minerals selenium and zinc. It is important to consider the correlation between nutrition and a healthy immune system (Chapter 3).

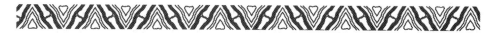

The exact cause of RA still continues to baffle experts. There is a school of thought which believes that a particular organism, *proteus*, which causes urinary tract infection, could be implicated. Most people who suffer from RA have certain genetic tissue that resembles the proteus bacterium. It is therefore thought that the immune system could possibly mistake the body tissue for proteus. This is further corroborated by the fact that that patients have higher than normal levels of antibodies to proteus in their blood. It may even explain the higher incidence of RA in women, as they are more prone to urinary tract infections.

Most arthritics, particularly those suffering from RA, also have food or chemical allergies and, again, environmental and dietary considerations are important. Exhaust fumes, gas and other chemicals all play a part in triggering and exacerbating the symptoms.

An imbalance of calcium may cause the bones to be porous and more prone to wear and tear. The balance of calcium is maintained by hormones. A whole host of factors, such as exposure to toxic substances, stress levels and consumption of alcohol, can contribute to the imbalance.

Treatment Of Rheumatism And Arthritis

Over 20 million prescriptions are written annually in the UK for *non-steroidal anti-inflammatory drugs* (NASAIDs) for the relief of arthritis. While these help in reducing stiffness and pain, they deal purely with suppressing the symptoms themselves and do not attack the root cause of many underlying problems. Additionally, their use is linked to gastric damage, internal bleeding and an increased incidence of food allergy. The long-term use of painkillers, such as *paracetamol*, is known to have a damaging effect upon the liver in particular. Yet, you do not have to grin and bear the discomfort of arthritis: there are a number of things you can do.

Your GP will probably be your first port of call, particularly if your arthritis is severe (Chapter 2). Herbal medicines can offer gentle, gradual improvement in your condition and they are largely free from side-effects (Chapter 4). Complementary therapies, such as aromatherapy, acupuncture and homoeopathy, also offer a drug-free solution (Chapters 5–8). Almost all complementary therapies aim to treat holistically, that is, the body, mind and spirit together, to get to the root of disease. However you decide to tackle your pain – with

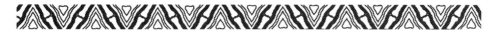

orthodox approaches alone, or with a combination of orthodox and complementary approaches, or with complementary approaches alone – you should be fully aware of the early warning signs. Your condition may be already long-standing and diagnosed, but you can help others to catch arthritis and rheumatism in their early stages.

Arthritis: Early Warning Signs

- Swelling, pain or tenderness in the joints
- Redness or warmth in a joint
- Early morning stiffness
- Difficulty or inability in moving a joint
- Note: the above symptoms should recur and last for two weeks or more.

Useful Addresses

Arthritis Care, 18 Stephenson Way, London NW1 2HD, Telephone: 071-916 1500, has an information/counselling service for arthritis and rheumatism sufferers on its main telephone number 10.00 AM – 4.00 PM on weekdays and a Freephone Helpline on 0800 289170 from 12.00 – 4.00 PM.

National Back Pain Association, 16 Elm Tree Road, Teddington, Middlesex TW11 8ST, Telephone: 081-977 5474, is an organisation working solely for back pain sufferers and their carers, funding research, teaching back care and encouraging self-help.

Repetitive Strain Injury, c/o Mr Mulelly, Chapel House, 152–156 High Street, Yiewsley, West Drayton. Middlesex UB7 7BD. Please send a SAE for information.

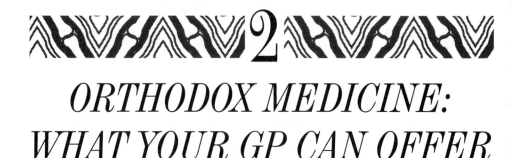

ORTHODOX MEDICINE: WHAT YOUR GP CAN OFFER

When we think of rheumatism we often picture a wizened elderly person with deformed joints who is crippled and unable to walk. It is frightening to imagine ourselves in the same position. Thankfully, such scenes are now uncommon in the West and the majority of people who suffer from joint problems and rheumatism are able to lead normal lives.

Rheumatism is, in fact, a vague term seldom used by doctors, except in the specific disorder rheumatoid arthritis. It is used here to cover a variety of conditions that do not involve joints but the structures around them, and only the most common are described below.

There are many forms of arthritis which are short-lived and which have a specific treatment, for example joint infections, although rare and serious, can be treated with *antibiotics* (substances used against bacterial infections). Diseases which affect joints and muscles can involve other parts of the body as well, such as the eye and the liver. Prompt diagnosis and treatment of these are essential to prevent serious damage. So it is important that anyone who has joint or severe muscle pains for more than a few days should seek the advice of their family doctor so that the cause can be investigated. Most of the time they will be reassured that there is not a serious cause for the problem.

Rheumatoid arthritis and osteoarthritis are the types of arthritis with which people are most familiar. Making a diagnosis, however, is sometimes difficult and it may be months or years before blood tests and other investigations show any definite disease. This may be difficult to accept at first but it is always possible to provide treatment while adopting a 'wait and see' policy. There is no cure for either of these chronic conditions and it takes some time to come to terms with this. Your own doctor is there to provide you with continuity of care, explanations and advice, as well as giving you access to other resources and providing initial treatment.

If you are acutely ill with joint pains or if other parts of your body are affected, such as the eye, referral to a specialist may be

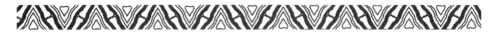

appropriate. Most people who have rheumatoid arthritis will be under the care of a consultant rheumatologist at some time.

In the early stages of an illness, there are always questions and worries which should be discussed with your doctor. Starting on tablet treatments or injections needs careful explanation of effects and side-effects and good communication between you and your doctor is likely to lessen unnecessary worry. Especially in the early stages of an illness, you may have a number of questions, and it can help to write a list of these to take with you to the surgery or outpatient clinic. Everyone deserves a clear explanation of their illness and this is a great help in motivating people to follow treatment correctly.

Someone with *progressive* (advancing in severity) arthritis that is disabling will need the care and attention of several members of the primary health care team, such as the district nurse or the physiotherapist, who may be attached to the GP's practice. Your doctor will be involved with liaising with these and other medical people, as well as the consultant rheumatologist.

Most people with long-standing joint problems will have regular visits to their family doctor for the monitoring of drug treatment and checking general well-being. The family doctor is in an ideal position to help you come to terms with what may be a long-standing illness and also with its possible effects on your family and relationships.

Below are the most common causes of arthritis and details of the types of treatment you can expect from your family doctor and specialist.

Rheumatoid Arthritis

Despite years of research, it is still unclear how this disorder commences. We do know that it is in some way connected with the immune system (see Chapter 1). There appears to be some influence on the disease from female hormones: about 60 per cent of women with RA notice an improvement during pregnancy. Unfortunately it is not yet known why.

Symptoms

RA may come on quite suddenly, with several joints becoming acutely swollen, stiff and painful overnight. The *metacarpo-phalangeal*

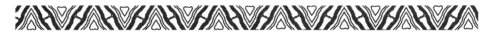

joints (joints in the hand) and the knuckles are commonly affected but any joint may be involved. Usually RA is ignored as 'just a touch of rheumatics' for weeks or months before help is sought – unfortunately giving the disorder time to gain hold. RA may also appear in a single joint, for example, the knee, and it then has to be differentiated from many other forms of arthritis, including infection and gout.

Complications

Many other parts of the body may be involved in the inflammatory process of rheumatoid disease. Commonly, the eye may be affected with insufficient lubrication. This is known as 'dry eye' syndrome and can be very uncomfortable. Artificial tears can help here. A serious complication is *iritis*, where the eye become acutely inflamed, red and often with haziness of vision. This needs urgent treatment with drops to *dilate* (widen) the pupil and steroid drops for the inflammation. It can be recurrent and needs to be monitored by a hospital specialist. There are many other possible complications that affect a minority of people. These include rupture of tendons, inflammation of blood vessels and kidney problems.

Diagnosis And Investigations

There are so many types of RA that it is not always possible for your GP to make a diagnosis straight away. Changes to the joints seen on X-ray do not occur until at least three months after the onset of symptoms, sometimes much longer, so you may not have this investigation immediately. Blood tests are usually helpful, though. One test you will almost certainly have is a full blood count which will check for *anaemia* (deficiency of red blood cells) and a test known as an *ESR* which stands for *erythrocyte sedimentation rate*. This test gives a rough idea of the amount of inflammation present in the body.

A more specific test can be done which looks for a substance called *rheumatoid factor*. This is a particular protein which is produced as part of the immune response, called *immunoglobulin M* (*IgM*) and which reacts with another protein called *immunoglobulin G* (*IgG*). The presence of this leads to the term *seropositive arthritis*, which applies to about 70 per cent of people with RA. Unfortunately, a few healthy people have it in their blood as well and a number of

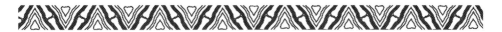

RA sufferers do *not* have it, so it is not always confirmatory. If rheumatoid factor is present, the amount can be measured and a high level is usually associated with a less-favourable outcome. More specialised blood tests may be needed to look for other antibodies in the blood. This will exclude some of the diseases related to RA, called the *collagen disorders.* An example of these is *systemic lupus erythematosus* which is described on page 36.

Outlook

Predicting the outcome for someone with RA is difficult because the course of the disease is extremely variable. About two-thirds of people remain reasonably well, and are able to lead perfectly normal lives or have only moderate disability. There are certain factors which make this outcome more likely, including, surprisingly, a sudden and severe onset. Remissions of the disease also indicate that the long-term outlook will be better and with less long-term disability than if there are unremitting symptoms. One-third of people, however, will have quite bad disability. Early indicators of this include nodules under the skin and changes on X-ray which show destruction of the joints. Involvement of other organs in the body, such as the lungs or liver, is also a poor sign.

Inheritance

When a family member is diagnosed as having RA, there is usually considerable worry as to whether it will be inherited. The likelihood of this happening is very small, in fact, though not easy to predict exactly. Studies on twins show that environmental factors are equally important. Certain *gene markers* have recently been discovered that are linked with RA and associated conditions. One of the gene markers is called HLA-DR4 but there are others. The presence of this, which is found by a special blood test, means that the person is more susceptible to RA but does not mean that he or she will inevitably suffer from it. More accurate assessment of risk will probably come in the future but, for now, the test is only performed rarely.

Physical Treatments

Specialists who may help you with exercises include the physiotherapist and occupational therapist. Some general practices have a physiotherapist who works for them at the surgery. Most people with moderate or severe arthritis, however, will probably be seen in a hospital environment where more specialised equipment and occupational therapy aids are available. *Hydrotherapy*, specialised exercises in a heated pool, should be available in your health region, but those of you in more rural areas may have to travel a long way to get it. A lot of patients find that their joints are much more mobile for a few days after the therapy but that they also feel utterly exhausted. It is wise to pace yourself carefully for this, and not plan too hectic a schedule afterwards.

Some very inflamed joints and tendons need to be rested and the physiotherapist will then supply you with splints. If the *cervical spine* (the bones in your neck) are affected you may be given a collar to wear in the short term. The aim of this is to give pain relief by flexing the head forwards slightly and stretching the neck to avoid pressure on the nerve roots which come out between the vertebral bones. There is a limit to the time that this should be worn, however, since overuse can lead to weakening of the neck muscles that support the spine. Neck exercises then become extremely important.

For chronic pain affecting the spine a device called a *TNS machine* may be used. This is a *transcutaneous nerve stimulator* which consists of a small box with electrodes that are placed on acupuncture points on the skin. Repeated electrical impulses are given which stimulate the nerves and block out painful sensation. Such stimulation may enable the body to produce its own pain-killing substances called *endorphins*. For reasons unknown, this treatment is very effective for some and not at all for others. Since it is virtually free of side-effects it is well worth a try; you can borrow or lease a TNS machine from your local physiotherapy department, reached via your GP.

Drug Treatments

For many years the drug of first choice for treating RA was simple aspirin, given in large doses. This has been almost completely superseded now by a related group of drugs called Non Steroid Anti-Inflammatory Drugs (NSAIDs) (see Chapter 1). This large group of drugs is used for a variety of disorders including injury to muscles and joints as well as many forms of arthritis.

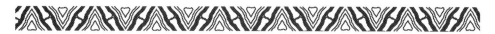

Most Commonly Used NSAIDs

Ibuprofen (trade name: Brufen)
Naproxen (trade name: Naprosyn)
Piroxicam (trade name: Feldene)
Mefenamic acid (trade name: Ponstan)
Diclofenac (trade name: Voltarol)
Fenoprofen (trade name: Fenopron)

Millions of prescriptions are given for NSAIDs every year and they account for a sizeable proportion of the average GP's drug budget. In the short term, they are relatively free of side-effects but anyone on long-term treatment should be monitored by their GP. They are drugs which alleviate the symptoms of stiffness, pain and swelling by blocking the production of substances called *prostaglandins*, which are responsible for producing inflammation. They do not alter the process of the disease nor do they affect the outlook but they do, undoubtedly, allow many sufferers to lead more normal lives than they would otherwise. The main side-effect is irritation of the lining of the stomach, which leads to indigestion, nausea and vomiting. If this happens to you, stop the tablets immediately and consult your doctor. A few patients who have had long-term treatment may develop stomach ulcers and these can sometimes bleed. This may lead to the person vomiting blood, which may look like coffee grounds if it has been partly digested, or to the passage of tarry stools. Again, consult you doctor immediately if this happens. These side-effects are less common when a NSAID is given in combination with an *H2 blocker drug*, for example, *Cimetidine*, which reduces the amount of acid in the stomach and protects the lining. This sort of combination is also available in one combined tablet.

Rare side-effects include suppression of the activity of bone marrow (which produces cells in the blood and factors which help clotting). This can lead to anaemia and problems of blood clotting and may be another reason why your blood should be checked if you take tablets long term.

Some NSAIDs are available as a gel to use locally and studies have shown that, taken like this, the drug is absorbed well into the bloodstream, so it can still affect the stomach lining. There is some doubt, therefore, that gels eliminate the incidence of side-effects. It is also likely that they are no more effective than tablets overall. Some drugs are available in *suppository* form (a solid for insertion into the rectum, vagina or urethra). This can be useful when taken at night-time to reduce stiffness in the morning, but the drug is also well absorbed into the bloodstream from the rectum so may still cause gastric symptoms. Occasionally, the injectable form of an NSAID may be used to relieve acute pain.

Second-line Drugs

When NSAIDs are inadequate to control symptoms and when the disease is obviously progressing, other drugs may be tried which may alter the disease process and so reduce the destruction to joints. These are virtually always started by the specialist but much of the day-to-day management and monitoring of their effect is done by the family doctor. Up to six months of treatment needs to be given to assess effectiveness.

Sulphasalazine (Trade Name: Salazopyirine)
This is a drug which is also used in inflammatory bowel conditions, such as *ulcerative colitis*. It is usually taken in tablet form and the dose increased over a number of weeks. Allergic reactions can occur, typically causing skin rashes, fever, nausea and indigestion, but otherwise it is relatively well tolerated. Over long periods of use it can cause suppression of the bone marrow and periodic blood tests are necessary to check for this.

Gold
This is usually given in injectable form after a test dose to check for allergy. The injections are given over a number of months or even years and the amount of gold gradually accumulates in the body. It is possibly one of the most effective second-line drugs if it can be tolerated. The tablet form of this treatment is now used less frequently as it seems less effective despite being better tolerated. Kidney function can be affected and blood and urine tests are needed regularly. Mouth ulcers may occur, in which case treatment must be stopped, and there are a number of other side-effects.

Penicillamine (Trade Name: Distamine)
A commonly used second-line tablet treatment that has been successful for a number of years and may be used if gold injections cannot be tolerated. It can take several months to have any effect and routine monitoring, as with the other drugs, is carried out. Skin rashes can be a problem.

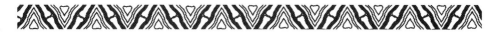

Hydroxychloroquine (Trade Name: Plaquenil)
Now seldom used, this drug is an anti-malarial which has many
potential side-effects but is tried if others are unsuccessful or cannot
be tolerated. Its main danger is damage to the *retina* (the sensitive
layer of the eye) so regular hospital check-ups are needed to guard
against this. Administered in tablet form, hydroxychloroquine does
not affect the blood so it can be useful for people who do not have
easy access to blood monitoring.

Third-line Drugs

Steroids
This class of drug has received a bad press in recent years because of
the wide variety of side-effects. The main tablet used is *prednisolone*
(trade name: Prednisone) which is often given in a coated form to
minimise stomach irritation. Only the most severe rheumatoid
patients are prescribed steroids nowadays, as there are other more
effective second-line treatments available. For those who cannot
tolerate second-line drugs, however, steroids can greatly reduce
discomfort and swelling of joints. They are sometimes used in high
doses initially then reduced to nothing over a period of a week or
more. However, some people who have a chronically active disease
need to stay on a small dose over the long term. Such people will
almost always be under the care of a rheumatologist as well as their
family doctor and are monitored to detect side-effects such as
thinning of the bones (*osteoporosis*) and diabetes. Weight gain can
also be a problem and needs to be addressed early to protect the
joints from excess strain.

   The use of steroid injections into joints is far less likely to cause
side-effects and can provide tremendous pain relief in single joints,
large and small. There is a very small risk, almost negligible, of
infection in the joint following this but it is otherwise extremely
helpful.

Azathioprine (Trade Name: Imuran)
Used also to suppress the immune system after organ transplants,
this is another drug that is thought to modify the disease process. It
may be given in addition to steroids and may reduce the need for
them. Potentially it has a lot of side-effects and not everyone can
tolerate it. Most importantly, it can cause suppression of the bone
marrow, so regular blood tests need to be taken. It comes in tablet

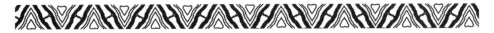

form and injections. Its effect may last for several weeks after it has been stopped.

Other Drugs

There are several other drugs which suppress the immune system and which are used in other serious diseases or following organ transplants. They are used only for rapidly progressive disease because they have potentially serious side-effects. Examples are *methotrexate, cyclophosphamide* and *chlorambucil.*

Surgery

Repair of tendons and replacement of diseased joints are now commonplace and successful procedures. Deciding when a joint should be replaced is usually a matter of consideration between the person concerned, their GP and the specialist, the orthopaedic surgeon. The amount of pain is an important factor as well as disability and deformity. Now even elbow and shoulder joints can be replaced, giving a new lease of life for many people.

General Advice And Self-help

While the commonest forms of arthritis have, as yet, no cure, there are still plenty of things you can do to help yourself. This includes taking the advice and guidance your own doctor will give you about your condition, taking your treatment correctly and being aware of possible side-effects.

Exercise

Taking as much exercise as possible is helpful in maintaining the flexibility of your joints and maintaining muscle strength – even if there is some pain, it is unlikely you will do lasting damage. Often swimming is a practical option since water supports the body's weight, allowing joints to be exercised in a different way and increasing mobility. However, if you have not exercised for some time or suffer from any other medical condition, it is wise to seek your GP's advice first.

Diet

A great deal of research has been done on the connection between diet and arthritis, into whether it can bring on the disease and

whether it affects its course. It seems that for some people, avoiding particular foods, such as dairy products and red meats, brings about an improvement in their arthritis (see Chapter 3). Particularly for RA, though, the nature of the illness is that it waxes and wanes and so proving benefit scientifically has not been possible so far. A diet which is plentiful in fresh fruit and vegetables, high in fibre and low in animal fat, is one which we should all follow, regardless of whether we have arthritis or not. It is this sort of healthy diet that protects us from heart disease, diabetes and some forms of cancer. In addition, a low-fat and high-fibre diet will keep your weight down and this is very important to minimise the stress and strain on joints. This is particularly important in OA of the knees, for example, because so much of the body's weight is taken on these joints when walking.

Claims that particular diets are helpful, for example, a diet consisting of a very restricted number of foods or a diet high in fish oil, are generally frowned upon by the medical profession, but some research results are encouraging. If in doubt, see your doctor who can recommend a dietician at the local hospital or one who may be working at the surgery.

Attitude

Being optimistic with a chronic illness is quite a challenge when the outlook is rather uncertain, especially if you have family commitments. However, we know that patients who are optimistic and who persevere with advice, treatment and exercise tend to fare better and to need less treatment with painkillers, than those who are pessimistic and inactive. There is increasing evidence now for the 'mind–body connection'. That is, if you have an image of yourself as well and healthy, this will influence your ability to cope with symptoms and it is possible that it may influence the outcome of the disease.

If you are one of those people who has a chronic form of arthritis, it can be difficult to have a positive attitude. There is often someone that you know who is severely disabled and who has not had the benefit of the more recent advances in treatment, to give a worrying picture. Building a positive image of yourself takes time and effort. Your own doctor is probably not the best person to help with this. After all, you tend to go to the doctor only when you are ill!

It is just such a task that can be helped along by complementary therapies. Having a realistic attitude to these in helping you to

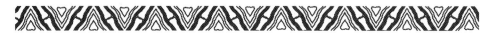

address your self-image is probably the best approach. No one has yet found a 'cure' for RA nor any of its associated conditions but complementary therapies help to make life more pleasant, and pain and stiffness less prominent as a result.

Depression

Any condition which is chronic can depress the sufferer, and the uncertainty of the outcome in RA in particular can cause some people to become clinically depressed. This is a common problem but it can come on very insidiously without you or your family recognising what is happening. There is a difference between being just 'down in the dumps' and having an illness which affects your mood, makes you weepy, unmotivated and sometimes inappropriately guilty. Sleep disturbance, loss of appetite and weight, and decreased sexual drive are all signs of depression that can easily be missed in someone with a chronic illness.

Tell your doctor if your mood is low or if you have any of these feelings. Anti-depressants tend to raise your pain threshold so you may not need so much in the way of painkillers or anti-inflammatory tablets. Anti-depressants are used commonly to help people who have chronic pain from a variety of causes and they work, even if the person does not appear to be depressed. You may not notice much difference for a few days, but 10 to 14 days after starting them, sleep patterns, appetite and mood do seem to improve for most people and pain decreases.

It may also be of value to have counselling either with a trained counsellor or psychologist, to whom your GP can refer you. Alternatively, one of the arthritis self-help groups can offer support from other sufferers or volunteer helpers, either individually or as part of a group. Their advice and information is invaluable.

The Collagen Diseases

There are a number of rare disorders which affect the connective tissue in the body, that is, the tissue which provides the strength in bones and ligaments. Examples are SLE, *dermatomyositis* and *scleroderma*. They are all potentially serious conditions that affect many parts of the body and are thought to be brought about by a defect in the immune system. They may all start with joint or muscle pains and can be detected with specific blood tests similar to the

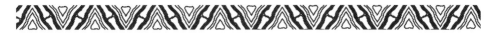

rheumatoid factor test for RA. Treatment varies between the conditions but because of their seriousness, steroid treatment is common and can be life saving. Diagnosis and treatment is mostly under the care of a rheumatologist but ongoing support and monitoring will be provided by your own doctor.

Osteoarthritis

Over the age of 65 about half the population have this condition to some degree, as studies of X-rays have shown. Not everyone, though, has symptoms (for these, see Chapter 1). The exact disease mechanism is unknown. Unlike RA there is little damage to the synovium but cartilage becomes damaged and the bone itself may become affected with formation of cysts. The joint becomes deformed so that there is loss of space between the joint surfaces, which rub together causing creaking and crunching noises. *Osteophytes* (bone spurs) may form. When this happens to the vertebrae in the neck it can cause entrapment of nerves, and pain may be referred to the shoulders and arms. Stiffness and deformity are the main problems of OA besides pain. The joints may become acutely inflamed but this is not common.

Like RA, there is a small hereditary component but environmental and other factors are more important in the development of the condition.

Diagnosis

There is no definitive test for OA and the diagnosis will usually be made by your doctor from the history you give and examination of the joints. There are characteristic changes on X-ray which have a different appearance from those seen in RA. There is usually loss of space visible between the two joint surfaces. In cases of doubt, testing for rheumatoid factor may be worthwhile.

Complications

It is the disability in hips and knees, that causes complications in managing everyday life. Some older people with multiple medical problems are not fit to have surgery performed and must live with their disability. The primary health care team may all then be involved to provide physiotherapy, occupational therapy, and

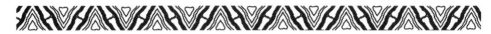

appropriate practical help to enable people to lead independent lives where possible. Simple aids, such as shoe raises and splints for knees and ankles, can make a big difference to mobility.

Treatment And General Measures

Keeping weight down and exercising are beneficial and there is increasing evidence that being fit and slim can help prevent the onset of OA.

Simple painkillers, such as paracetamol and aspirin, are adequate for many people with mild disease; the anti-inflammatory drugs described above can give greater relief but these do not alter the degenerative process. There has been some research to suggest that there is a repair component to the disease which gives hope for future development of a drug that may halt or at least slow down joint destruction. As with RA, steroid injections into joints can give excellent pain relief. Beyond drugs, the only orthodox resort to relieve pain and stiffness is replacement of joints. Because of a rise in the number of pensioners, the demand for joint replacements has steadily increased in the last few decades. There is also the increased expectation of a good quality of life that rightly causes patients to request specialist referral for this. How these increasing demands are to be met in the future is one of the many dilemmas that now faces the NHS in Britain and all health systems in the Western world.

Gout

We usually think of gout as a disease of older men but it can occur in women, although less commonly. It is caused by *hyperuricaemia,* an excess of uric acid in the blood which becomes deposited in the joints in crystal form. These crystals initiate an acute inflammatory reaction which can cause severe pain. The joint becomes hot and swollen and extremely tender to the touch. Any joint in the body may be affected, and if not treated over several years, crystals may be deposited in the kidney, causing permanent damage. About 20 per cent of people with chronic gout, now relatively unusual, develop *tophi,* which are solid lumps of uric acid around the joints and in the skin, usually over the ear. Chronic gout causes joint destruction and secondary osteoarthritis. The acute condition can be precipitated by too much alcohol as well as by certain foods, such as herring, yeast extract and red meat.

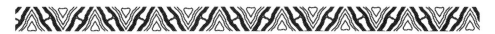

Diagnosis

This may be obvious just on examination by your own doctor, especially if you have suffered from it before, but there are several causes of acutely swollen joints that need to be excluded. Amongst these are various infective causes and a condition called *pseudo-gout* where the crystals consist of a chemical called *pyrophosphate*. This usually occurs in people over 55 and is most common in the knee.

Diagnosing gout is usually easy from the history and the site of joint pain. A blood test will confirm a raised level of uric acid. Problems can arise, however, as the uric acid level is sometimes raised in people who are entirely free from joint symptoms. Sometimes the only way to be certain is to take a sample of synovial fluid from the joint with a needle and examine it microscopically. The crystals can then be identified and differentiated from pyrophosphate. If no crystals are present, it is possible that the joint is infected. This needs prompt treatment, so if a joint becomes suddenly inflamed and you feel ill generally, you should see a doctor urgently.

Diet

Purine is the substance which is broken down to uric acid in the body and there are many foods which contain it in large amounts. Cutting them out and reducing or stopping alcohol may prevent gout in some individuals. The need for dietary control has lessened a great deal since allopurinol became available, but diet should not be ignored. In general health terms, a diet that is low in animal fat, high in fibre and full of fresh fruit and vegetables is likely to prevent illness and promote longevity.

Treatment

Painkillers

Ordinary paracetamol or aspirin are sometimes enough for a mild attack of gout but most people need something stronger. Combinations of paracetamol with codeine are also available over-the-counter.

NSAIDs

These drugs are the most commonly prescribed for an acute episode as they reduce joint inflammation. They are described fully under the treatment of rheumatoid arthritis.

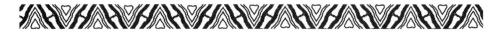

Colchicine

One of the older treatments, this drug is effective for an acute attack. The dose has to be increased gradually. It is suitable for those people who get severe side-effects from NSAIDs or who have a past history of stomach ulcers. It is seldom used now for prevention of attacks since allopurinol became available. Side-effects are relatively uncommon but may include nausea, vomiting and rashes. Care must be taken when other medicines are prescribed as it can, for example, increase the effect of sedatives.

Allopurinol (Zyloric)

Given as a once daily tablet, this drug will prevent gout completely in many people and is the standard prophylactic treatment. It acts by stopping the formation of uric acid crystals in the joints. It is not effective in an acute attack and in the first few months of treatment can increase the episodes of gout, so it is often given with an anti-inflammatory drug initially.   Although it is generally well tolerated, it may cause a rash or nausea and, rarely, tingling in the hands and feet. If these symptoms occur, it should be stopped.

Probenecid

This drug works by increasing the amount of uric acid in the urine and, like allopurinol, is not effective in an acute attack. It comes in tablet form and is sometimes given to increase the effect of certain antibiotics. Because it acts on the kidney, it can increase the risk of uric acid kidney stones. It also interacts with a large number of other drugs and for this reason it is not now prescribed very often.

Ankylosing Spondylitis And Related Disorders

There are a number of conditions which have features in common and which are known in the medical world as *seronegative spondylarthritides*. Examples of these are ankylosing spondylitis, psoriatic arthropathy, arthritis associated with ulcerative colitis and Reiter's syndrome. These 'overlap' to some extent in that the presence of one makes it more likely for another of the group to develop in an individual. They all have a small hereditary tendency. A particular genetic marker is present in a proportion of affected individuals and it gives some idea of the risk of developing any of the conditions. This marker is called *HLA B27*. The word *seronegative*

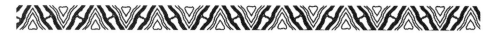

means that the blood test for rheumatoid factor is negative.

Reiter's Syndrome

This condition is a collection of symptoms comprising *urethritis*, which causes pain on passing urine, *conjunctivitis*, causing redness of the eye and *arthritis*, affecting only a few joints at a time. It is common in young men and is sometimes associated with sexually transmitted disease, particularly the germ *chlamydia*, so excluding and treating any infection of this nature is most important. Reiter's syndrome can become a chronic and relapsing condition and is treated symptomatically with anti-inflammatory drugs.

Ankylosing Spondylitis

This is predominantly a disease of young men which involves the lower spine and part of the pelvis. It has a marked hereditary tendency and is associated with HLA B27 more strongly than the other diseases. Inflammation of the spine can lead to complete fusion of the lower vertebrae if it is not diagnosed. Inflammation of the eye can also occur, called *iritis*. This needs careful treatment and follow-up by an eye specialist to avoid permanent damage in the eye.

The most important aspect of treatment is maintaining the flexibility of the spine with a relentless routine of daily exercises and extra physiotherapy where necessary. Many people take daily NSAIDs at night-time to alleviate stiffness of the spine in the mornings.

Polymyalgia Rheumatica

No one knows what causes this disease which affects people over 50 almost exclusively. The main features are pain and stiffness in the upper part of the limbs often with tenderness of the muscles of the upper arm. There may be generalised illness with loss of appetite and weight, as well as a tendency to depression. It may sometimes be associated with an inflammation of the main artery running over the temples, the *temporal artery*. If left untreated, this can cause sudden blindness, so any severe headache in this region should be promptly investigated by your doctor. There is no specific test for the condition but the test called the *ESR*, explained earlier, is substantially raised. Samples of the temporal artery can be examined

microscopically for changes of inflammation. When polymyalgia is present alone, small doses of oral steroids and NSAIDs are usually enough to control symptoms. Temporal arteritis, however, is such a dangerous condition to the eye that high doses of steroids are required initially until the ESR level falls and they can then be carefully reduced. Some people need to stay on them in the long term.

Arthritis In Children

We do not usually associate arthritis with the young but it is not a rare occurrence by any means. Viral illnesses such as *rubella*, known commonly as German measles, can cause swelling of the joints which may last for several weeks after the initial illness before it finally disappears; other viruses may cause a similar picture in children and adults alike. Acute bacterial infection in a joint is fairly unusual but serious in children and most often occurs in the upper limb bones, the humerus and femur. The child can become very ill if germs escape from the infected joint into the bloodstream, so it is important that any child with one or more swollen joints is seen straightaway by a doctor.

There are several types of arthritis in children, of unknown origin, which are classified in the medical world by the way in which they start. The group name for them is *juvenile chronic arthritis*. If there are only one or two joints involved at the onset but with fever and a rash, the illness is called *Still's disease*, after the doctor from Great Ormond Street Hospital who linked all the symptoms together. Arthritis may occur without generalised illness as well in a few or many joints. The deformity of joints tends to be less than in adults. How these children are investigated depends on how ill they are when seen by the doctor. It is important to exclude joint infection first with blood tests and X-rays and this may need hospital admission. Almost all but the mildest of problems will need the expertise of a consultant paediatrician or children's rheumatologist. Investigations are likely to include blood tests like the ESR and the test for anaemia. The rheumatoid factor is likely to be negative in most children, except for some teenage girls who have an illness similar in pattern to RA.

Treatment is often difficult because of generalised illness, and although NSAIDs are given to most children, the disease may need oral steroid treatment as well at some time to get it under control.

The main problem with this is the potential stunting of growth that may occur, and careful monitoring is necessary. There have been a number of trials in children with the second- and third-line drugs described previously for rheumatoid arthritis and *methotrexate* has shown some promise, but is not commonly used as yet. All the treatments for RA may be offered to children and injection of joints with steroids can be particularly helpful in restoring mobility.

Outlook

Juvenile chronic arthritis is a group of diseases and predicting the outcome is therefore difficult. We do know, however, that where few joints are involved, there is a 50 per cent chance that the child will get better spontaneously. A significant number continue with joint inflammation into adulthood, but their deformity tends to be less than with adult onset disease. There are a number of genetic markers that can predict the outcome to some extent. For example, boys with the HLA B27 marker have a 20 per cent chance of developing ankylosing spondylitis in adulthood.

Support and explanation of treatment of juvenile arthritis are the main functions of the family doctor, as well as monitoring for side-effects and communicating parents' questions and worries to the specialist where appropriate.

Some common and important causes of arthritis have been explained here but there are many types of joint and muscle pain that defy a full diagnosis. Aches and pains in the lumbar region and in the neck and shoulders are common and will often be related to poor posture, overweight or lack of fitness. Don't be surprised if your doctor gives you general advice to lose weight and become more active, instead of a prescription. The commonly prescribed NSAIDs can only do so much. Consulting an alternative practitioner may be helpful once it is clear that there is not a serious underlying cause for the problem but you should always tell your GP if this is what you intend and make sure that the practitioner concerned has appropriate qualifications.

NUTRITION: FOOD FOR HEALTHY JOINTS

The science of nutrition has come a long way in the last hundred years and has evolved through several stages. Initially, diseases such as scurvy and pellagra were recognised as *deficiency diseases* (their cause is due to a lack of essential nutrients). The link between food and health thus established, deficiency diseases were easily eliminated by the simple expedient of including the missing nutrients in the diet. In this way, the concept of a well-balanced diet (one that prevented the onset of disease) gained currency.

Later, the role of nutrition expanded from treatment of illnesses to their prevention. Research showed that there was a strong relationship between the dietary intake of nutrients and the development, progression and cure of diseases other than deficiency diseases. Further research uncovered the impact of nutrition on the immune system, and the possible prevention of cancers, heart disease and diseases such as arthritis and osteoporosis.

Improving the quality of the diet and introducing immune-boosting supplementation can help reduce pain and inflammation. Furthermore, they can also mitigate the adverse effects of some drugs. However, before we can consider the various dietary factors, it is important to consider the link between immune-related degenerative diseases – twentieth-century ailments – and our diet. It is now accepted amongst nutritionists that a contributory factor to modern diseases is a result of not following a diet that provides us with the correct nutrients.

A World Health Organisation report recommends a daily intake of 400 g (1 lb) of fruit and vegetables to include pulses, seeds and nuts for optimal health. The report also underlines the fact that a typical western diet lacks sufficient quantities of essential nutrients and that we may be overfed but still remain undernourished. It must be understood, however, that nutritional therapy does not offer magic pills or potions to cure or prevent specific ailments.

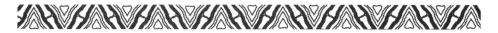

Nutrients And Food

We all need nutrients in their correct amounts for positive, glowing, good health. What, though, are these amounts? A pregnant woman, for example, has increased dietary needs in order to nourish her unborn child; adolescents require greater quantities of certain nutrients to ensure full growth and development; the elderly need extra nutrients to counteract the effects of ageing; whilst a busy executive needs increased amounts of particular nutrients to offset the damaging effects of stress. Just as an athlete requires more calories than a sedentary office worker, so do their nutrient intakes differ: even the basic difference between the sexes, regardless of age and other factors, results in a different set of nutrient requirements.

There are reasons for thinking that we may not be getting all the nourishment we need from our food, even if we are making the right food choices. It is important to realise that vitamins cannot be manufactured by the body and must therefore come from the diet. Nature has packed unprocessed foods with the vitamins we need, but vitamins are delicate, unstable entities that can easily be destroyed during the many processing methods used in modern food production. In its progress from farm to factory to supermarket, food is depleted of essential vitamins and minerals. Whatever goodness remains is quite probably lost between the freezer and microwave before its final arrival on the plate. You may be eating up your greens, but are they providing you with any goodness?

Dietary Considerations

The first and foremost consideration for healthy bones and joints is to enjoy a diet that is low in fats, high in fibre and that has adequate levels of vitamins and minerals. A good diet should contain a variety of fresh fruit and vegetables, wholegrain breads, cereals, beans and pulses with small amounts of lean meats, chicken and fish (the diet should not be excessive in protein). Care must be taken to avoid obesity and overweight – this is particularly vital for arthritics.

Where there is a deficiency of certain nutrients, supplements in the form of pills, capsules or liquids may be taken in consultation with a qualified nutritionist or a dietary therapist. This will ensure that the correct balances between nutrients are maintained.

Guidelines For Healthy Eating

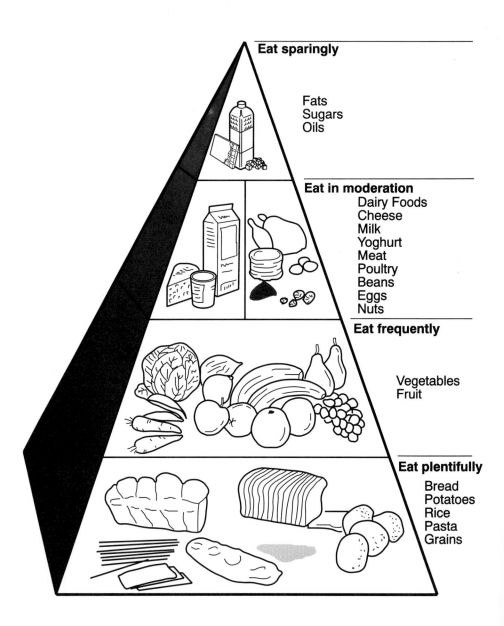

Eat sparingly

Fats
Sugars
Oils

Eat in moderation
Dairy Foods
Cheese
Milk
Yoghurt
Meat
Poultry
Beans
Eggs
Nuts

Eat frequently

Vegetables
Fruit

Eat plentifully

Bread
Potatoes
Rice
Pasta
Grains

The Healthy Eating Pyramid was evolved by nutritionists in the US. It has been adapted by the Dunn Nutritional Centre for application in Britain. It shows very clearly which foods we should be eating in large quantities and which we should be eating in only small amounts.

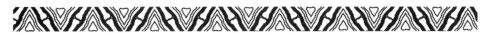

Vitamins and minerals work together in interrelated systems in the body. For example, both vitamin D and magnesium are necessary for the proper utilisation of calcium. Vitamin C is necessary for iron absorption and vitamin E protects vitamins A and D from oxidation. Some nutrients taken on their own deplete others, for example, large quantities of zinc can cause a depletion of copper and can exacerbate existing ailments. The haphazard taking of supplements can be wasteful, inefficient and may even cause deficiency of other nutrients, creating an imbalance in the entire system.

Drugs sometimes cause dietary deficiencies either by destroying nutrients or by using them up. A nutritional counsellor will consider drug interactions and nutritional deficiencies and will suggest a carefully balanced supplements programme.

Acid/Alkali Balance And Inflammation

The acid/alkali food balance is highly significant in inflammatory conditions. Acid-forming foods are meat, fish, most cereals, most nuts and dairy foods. Most fruits and vegetables, except citrus fruits and tomatoes, are alkali-forming foods.

For arthritis, a diet that is predominantly alkaline would help in reducing inflammation. While most experts recognise the different dietary needs of each individual, generally, a diet consisting of 80 per cent alkali-forming foods and 20 per cent acid-forming foods is considered an ideal balance. For a detailed dietary recommendation, see *Arthritis, Rheumatism &Psoriasis* by Jan De Vries (Mainstream Publishing).

Antioxidant Nutrients

We saw in Chapter 1 the damage free radicals can do – but we can protect ourselves from free radicals by increasing our intake of *antioxidants.* Increased intake of antioxidant nutrients reduces free radical damage to joint linings. It is this damage that results in the accumulation of fluids and subsequent swelling and pain experienced by RA sufferers.The antioxidant nutrients therefore play an important role in reducing inflammation and in boosting the immune system.

Vitamin C
Vitamin C is perhaps the most researched antioxidant substance.

Ascorbic acid, to use vitamin C's scientific name, is soluble in water and provides antioxidant protection for the watery compartments of our cells, tissues and organs. Our bodies cannot make our own vitamin C so we are dependent upon food sources of this vital nutrient.

With specific reference to arthritis, vitamin C is also important for both bone and cartilage formation and hence healthy joints. *Collagen,* the building material for bone and cartilage, needs vitamin C for its formation.

Vitamin C is found in citrus fruit, green vegetables, potatoes and fruit juice, so an adequate consumption of these foods will go a long way towards boosting the immune system.

Vitamin E

Alpha-tocopherol, to give vitamin E its other name, is a powerful nutrient which, in common with many other nutrients, plays a crucial role in overall health. It increases the oxygen supply to muscles by improving the circulation and so increases exercise capacity.

As an antioxidant, vitamin E has a myriad of vital functions. It stabilises membranes and protects them against free radical damage, protects the eyes, skin, liver, breast and calf muscle tissues and protects and increases the body's store of vitamin A. Vitamin E is enhanced by other antioxidants, such as vitamin C and the mineral selenium.

Foods rich in vitamin E include cold-pressed oils (wheatgerm, safflower, sunflower and soybean), nuts and seeds, wheatgerm, asparagus, spinach, broccoli, butter, bananas and strawberries.

Vitamin A

Vitamin A is found in eggs, milk, lamb's liver, halibut liver oil, cod liver oil, dairy products, pig's kidney, beef, mackerel and canned sardines.

Zinc

Zinc is found in *alpha-macroglobulin,* an important protein in the body's immune system, so it stands to reason that a shortage of this mineral will severely affect the body's defence against disease. Additionally, zinc can help to clear certain toxic metals from the body (typically, cadmium and lead which are present in car exhaust fumes), thus further helping the immune system.

Zinc is also essential for normal cell division and function, so it

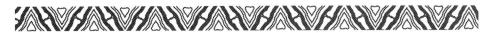

plays a part in protecting the cells in addition to its antioxidant activities. As part of the antioxidant enzyme *superoxide dismutase* (*SOD*) zinc influences inflammation and is particularly active with iron in the synovial fluid of arthritics.

Zinc is present in dairy products, beef, chicken, white fish and bread. It is an all-round valuable nutrient – so make sure your intake is satisfactory. A common sign of zinc deficiency is white marks on the fingernails.

Selenium

Its name derived from the Greek goddess of the moon, Selene, this antioxidant trace mineral was first regarded as a poison until the discovery that it was needed to prevent degeneration of the liver tissue. In addition to its role as an antioxidant in its own right, selenium serves as a mineral cofactor in the enzyme *glutathione peroxide*. This enzyme is important in reducing the production of inflammatory *prostaglandins*.

Iron

In addition to its role in helping to carry oxygen to the cells, iron is also needed for the antioxidant enzyme SOD to function. Hence, it is important in inflammatory conditions such as arthritis. Like zinc, the iron levels in the synovial fluids of arthritics are higher, which indicates an increased activity against joint damage.

Calcium And Magnesium

The most abundant mineral in the body, 99 per cent of calcium is present in the bones and teeth. However, the one per cent present in the muscles, nerves and the bloodstream plays a vital role in a number of enzymes. For proper calcium use, magnesium is also required, as is vitamin D for absorption.

Fish Oils

RA patients report improvements in morning stiffness when they take fish oil capsules. Folk medicine in many countries recommends 'oiling creaking joints' with fish oil. The idea that fish oils somehow help 'lubricate' joints (like rusty door hinges) is fallacious – it has no effect at all.

Clinical tests show that fish oil extracts treat arthritis effectively. A product combining fish oils with evening primrose oil used in a large trial organised by orthopaedic specialists involving hundreds

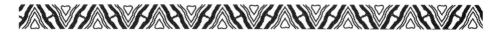

of RA sufferers was found to be sufficiently effective to allow a large number of patients to reduce the doses of their antiarthritic drugs – a vivid illustration of the replacement of drugs with a natural substance free from side-effects.

The special fatty acids in fish oils are known as *eicosapentaenoic acid* (*EPA*) and *docosahexaenoic acid* (*DHA*). These can convert into anti-inflammatory substances easing the joint pain and stiffness.

Most people associate fish oils with cod liver oil. For centuries cod liver oil has been used as a preventative against winter ills. In 1752 Dr Samuel Kay, at Manchester Infirmary, used cod liver oil to treat rheumatic pain and bone disorders. Physicians in the Victorian era used cod liver oil to treat gout, consumption, bronchitis, chronic skin diseases and rickets. While the doctors of the time accepted that cod liver oil was effective, no one knew why it was so. It was not until the discovery of vitamins in 1912 that scientists began to understand how and why cod liver oil was of benefit to human health.

It was then found to be one of the richest sources of vitamins A and D. By now it had been established that both these vitamins were needed for healthy skin, teeth and bones. It was realised that the reason why cod liver oil was so effective against rickets (the debilitating childhood bone disease) was that it provided vitamin D, a lack of which caused the disease. During the Industrial Revolution rickets was common among the children of workers, who spent much of their lives working in appalling conditions.

Because of these discoveries, cod liver oil was regarded as a major player in the growth and development of children. Rickets is normally thought of as a disease of the past. But even today, the Department of Health has mounted a campaign to make Asian parents more aware of the risks of rickets and has in fact advocated the use of cod liver oil. In addition to obtaining vitamin D from our diet, we also synthesise it through our skin when exposed to sunlight. Fair skinned people can synthesise this vitamin but people with dark skins find it more difficult to absorb sufficient sunlight necessary to make vitamin D.

It was not until the 1970s that scientists realised that there was more to fish oils than cod liver oil. Studies of the Greenland Eskimos discovered that, despite a diet high in animal fat and protein and low in fibre, the Eskimos had a very low incidence of heart disease and RA compared to the rest of the Western world.

Two Danish scientists, John Dyerberg and Hans Bang, took

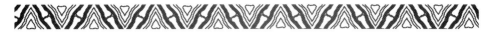

samples of Eskimo blood during a journey to Greenland in 1976 when they accompanied Dr Hugh Sinclair, a nutritional biochemist who first showed that Eskimos have very low blood cholesterol levels despite a diet which includes the highest animal fat content of any diet in the world.

When Dyerberg and Bang analysed the fats in Eskimos' blood, they found that it contained a very high level of the essential fatty acids EPA and DHA. As a result there has been consistent interest in the subject and a number of research papers have been published in medical journals pointing to a connection between these *omega-3* fatty acids and heart disease. In particular the EPA content is found to have been most effective in lowering the total blood cholesterol and *LDL (Low Density Lipoprotein)*, and increasing the *HDL (High Density Lipoprotein)* content. At last the magic ingredient behind the generally accepted belief that fish is good for us, was discovered.

Though its name sounds like something from science fiction, omega-3 is far from fictional. It is a name given to a group of essential fatty acids which are derived primarily from oily fish, such as mackerel, salmon and herring. They are called 'essential' because the body cannot manufacture them and they must come from the diet.

Fish oil concentrates have been shown to reduce the symptoms of swollen and tender joints, morning stiffness and pain in sufferers of RA. It is thought that fish oils work by suppressing production of two molecules called *leukotriene B4* (known for its powerful inflammatory properties) and *interleukin-1* (which is involved in the breakdown of cartilage and loss of appetite associated with RA).

Today fish consumption in this country is at its lowest ever – particularly consumption of fish which are a primary dietary source of omega-3 essential fatty acids. One of the simplest steps we can take to protect our health is to increase our consumption of the following fish (all rich in omega-3 fatty acids):

- mackerel;
- herrings;
- sardines;
- tuna (fresh);
- lake trout;
- salmon.

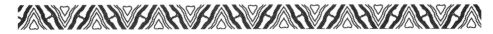

Evening Primrose Oil

Most vegetable oils contain linoleic acid which is an essential fatty acid. The normal diet is quite sufficient in linoleic acid. However, before this essential fatty acid can be used by the body, it has to be converted to a hormone-like substance called *prostaglandin PGE1*. Depending upon their type, some prostaglandins encourage inflammation while others reduce it. PGE1 is an anti-inflammatory prostaglandin. The conversion from linoleic acid to PGE1 is in stages. First, the linoleic acid from vegetable oils is converted into *gamma linolenic acid* (*GLA*) and then to *di-homo gammalinolenic acid* (*DGLA*) and then to PGE1. Unfortunately, this conversion is fraught with difficulties and can easily be blocked by a whole host of factors. Viruses, cholesterol, saturated fatty acids, alcohol, insufficient insulin, radiation, vitamin and mineral deficiency and the ageing process all contribute to blocking or adversely affecting this conversion.

Evening primrose oil has an unusually high amount of GLA and therefore it can help surmount all these blockages. Such a source of dietary GLA can therefore be extremely valuable since it can provide the material from which prostaglandin E1 can easily be produced. Recent studies indicate that evening primrose oil can ease the pain and stiffness of RA. Evening primrose oil is also known to help regulate the immune system so that it can better differentiate between 'self' and 'non-self' (see Chapter 1). Hence it helps deal with autoimmune diseases such as RA, where the immune system is overactive and appears to attack the joints. When it is mixed with fish oils even better results are obtained.

Superoxide Dismutase (SOD)

SOD is an enzyme reputed to rout out free radicals. SOD is produced naturally in the body in the nuclei of cells, but sometimes not enough SOD is produced. Hence some heavy smokers, who are producing enough SOD to destroy free radicals, can escape without falling prey to cancer, while others may smoke less but do contract cancer. Supplementation with SOD can strengthen the body's immune system and lessen chances of developing immune-related diseases.

Tests can be undertaken to establish existing levels of SOD and research is under way to predict how levels will perform. SOD has

the ability to reduce *lipid peroxides* (heavy-duty free radicals which have a long life and are extremely harmful if present in excess).

SOD is taken either via injections, when it has been shown to be of benefit to sufferers of severe RA, or via tablets. Unfortunately, while tablets are more suitable for general widespread use, when the tablet is swallowed SOD is probably for the most part broken down through the digestive process and therefore rendered inactive. A new process has been developed which is reputed to keep the drug active, but in general it would seem that, for the time being, SOD must remain in somewhat restricted use.

Shark Cartilage And Green Lipped Mussel

A somewhat gruesome nutrient, shark cartilage, has been used in scientific research to relieve arthritic symptoms. Shark cartilage stops the growth of cancer cells by inhibiting the cells' blood supply; this process is called *anti-angiogenesis*. A Belgian vet has also found success when treating dogs with OA with shark cartilage. However, shark cartilage is a relatively new discovery and is not widely available, nor is there a proliferation of scientific research into its effects. It could be argued that, even if it works, it is environmentally unfriendly.

Green lipped mussel extract originates from New Zealand where it has been used by the Maoris for centuries as a cure for many ills. The anti-inflammatory properties of the green lipped mussel are extracted from the gonads of the mussel and its effects on reducing swellings and inflammations has been documented for some decades. Sufferers of arthritis tend to experience some improvement in their condition after six months continued dosage of the green lipped mussel extract. Although extensive studies have not yet discovered an explanation for the therapeutic value of the mussel, its success rate is attested by many.

Nutritional Considerations

- All the antioxidant nutrients, such as zinc, selenium and vitamins A, C and E are important aspects in any immune system disorder.
- Those who cannot take regular exercise are more vulnerable to calcium loss from the bones (see 'Anti-Arthritis Exercise' on page 56). RA sufferers are likely to benefit from taking additional calcium with magnesium.

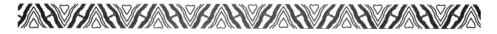

- In RA frequently there is an imbalance of hydrochloric acid, digestive pain and poor absorption. Digestive enzymes are helpful.
- Special fats known as *omega-6*, found in evening primrose oil, are of benefit .
- Fish oil is thought to be the most effective source of omega-3, another special fat which is even less common in the diet than omega-6 .

Dietary Recommendations For Osteoarthritis

- Low sugar intake.
- Low-fat diet of unsaturated fats.
- The supplements listed for RA may be beneficial (see page 55). In addition, calcium and magnesium are recommended, especially for younger people.

Therapeutic Foods

- Sesame seeds, artichokes, green beans, millet, celery, barley, okra, almonds, turnip greens, raw goat's milk, cherries, pineapple, watercress, blackberries, blackcurrants, limes, lettuce and olive oil.

Foods To Avoid

- Animal products, cow's milk and other dairy products, as they contain substances that might promote inflammation.
- Spinach, asparagus, rhubarb, vegetables from the nightshade family, (tomatoes, green peppers, potatoes, pimentoes, eggplant, tobacco), coffee, caffeine, sugar, refined foods and fried foods.

Dietary Recommendations For Rheumatoid Arthritis

- Low sugar intake.
- Low-fat diet of unsaturated fats.

Therapeutic Foods

- Increase omega-3 and omega-6 fatty acids: vegetable, nut, seed oils, salmon, herring, mackerel, sardines, walnuts and evening primrose oil.

- Sesame seeds, artichokes, green beans, millet, celery, barley, okra, almonds, turnip greens,cherries, pineapple, watercress, blackberries, blackcurrants, limes, lettuce and olive oil.
- Fresh juices: celery and parsley, cucumber, endive, apple and grapefruit.

Foods To Avoid

- Animal products, cow's milk and other dairy products due to the promotion of PGE2 pro-inflammatory mediators.
- Spinach, asparagus, rhubarb, vegetables from the nightshade family, (tomatoes, green peppers, potatoes, pimentoes, eggplant, tobacco), coffee, caffeine, sugar, refined foods, fried foods.

Supplements

- Broad-based, one-a-day multivitamin mineral preparation.
- Vitamin C 1000 mg per day. (Possibly buffered)
- Vitamin E 400 iu per day.
- Evening primrose oil 2 to 3 g per day.
- Fish oil 3 to 4 g per day.

Nutrition: Fundamental To Any Form Of Therapy

Most orthodox and complementary practitioners will tell you that underlying all disease is the breakdown of the body's natural functions. Poor nutrition is one of the primary causes of breakdown.

Hippocrates, the 'father of medicine', recognised this 2,000 years ago. Yet his words, 'Let food be your medicine, and your medicine be your food', seem to have been forgotten by modern medicine.

Of course, there is no doubt that our current sophisticated knowledge of the disease process has led to the production of specific drugs to counteract the symptoms of arthritis. But these drugs are often of only short-term benefit. They may help to relieve the symptoms but they do not prevent them from recurring. A return to basics, to food as medicine, can surely help.

It is only just emerging that changes in lifestyle and eating habits during the last 100 years have heaped an untold burden on our bodies. The body, through its immune system, has an amazing capacity to deal with the viruses, bacteria and other organisms that are an integral part of our lives. However, lack of nutrients, as we

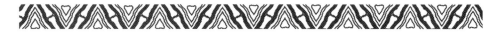

have seen, can weaken the immune system and impair its function leading to a whole host of degenerative diseases. To understand this is to understand the role of nutrition in the prevention of rheumatism and arthritis.

Anti-Arthritis Exercise

Exercise keeps the joints moving and lessens the opportunity for them to seize up. Strengthening exercises increase bone density and retain the calcium content of the bones, although this needs to be done regularly to maintain the effect. Overtraining, however, is damaging and can even depress the immune system.

Careful, regular exercise not only maintains or improves bone density, it also keeps the muscles loose and relaxed and works the *cardiovascular system* (heart and blood vessels), thereby ensuring the efficient blood supply to all parts of the body. Furthermore, exercise improves stamina, relaxes the mind and promotes good sleep. Endorphins are released during exercise, which is why we tend to feel happier after exercising. The benefits of exercise, then, are irrefutable for everyone, but which type of exercise is best for arthritis sufferers?

Swimming is best for arthritics since water supports the body, encourages suppleness, stimulates cardiovascular action and gets the muscles and cartilage working. It is gentle in that it does not place stress on parts of the body in the way that jogging, squash and aerobics do. Gardening is good to build up strength, while a brisk walk will get the circulation, muscles and joints all working.

Establish an exercise routine and keep to it. Try to swim, walk, garden or do some yoga or Tai Chi every day, even if it is only for 15 minutes. A little exercise every day will benefit you far more than a massive exercise session twice a week. Be careful not to overdo it – if you feel pain, even two hours after you have ceased to exercise, do a little less next time.

Finding A Nutrition Therapist

Dietitians can be consulted free via your GP, as there is one in every district, usually based at the main hospital. Many are keen to help people improve their eating habits. Or, for a list of practitioners or further information write, enclosing a SAE to:

The British Naturopathic and Osteopathic Association, 6 Netherall Gardens, London NW3 5RR;

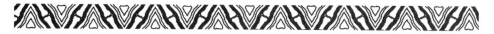

The British Society for Nutritional Medicine, 4 Museum Street, York, YO1 2ES;

The Nutrition Association, 36 Wycombe Road, Marlow, Buckinghamshire SL7 3HX.

Further Reading

Arthritis, Rheumatism and Psoriasis by Jan De Vries (Mainstream Publishing)
Say No To Arthritis by Patrick Holford (ION Press)
Tai Chi: Headway Lifeguides by Robert Parry (Headway)
The Eskimo Diet by R. Saynor and L. Ryan (Ebury Press)
Vitamin Guide by Hasnain Walji (Element Books)
Vitamins, Minerals and Dietary Supplements: A Definitive Guide to Healthy Eating, by Hasnain Walji (Headway, October 1994)
Yoga: Headway Lifeguides by Mary Stewart (Headway)

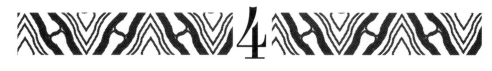

HERBALISM: NATURE'S PHARMACY

Conventional medicine developed out of herbal medicine. Many of today's chemical drugs are synthetic recreations of traditional herbal remedies: the active ingredient in black willow, for example, is aspirin, while steroids are based on the chemical recreation of the active ingredient found in the Mexican wild yam. So conventional medicine recognises the effectiveness of herbalism. The World Health Organisation estimates that herbalism is the most widely practised form of healing in the whole world. Yet in the nineteenth century the National Association (later to become the Institute) of Medical Herbalists was founded in the face of conventional medical practice which sought to ban the practice of herbalism.

Today, the combination of disillusionment with modern drugs because of their side-effects, together with a growing awareness of the environment and our place in it, has led to a resurgence in the West of traditional, ancient remedies. Herbalism is enjoying renewed interest and support because a growing number of Westerners are finding that it works, and works without dangerous side-effects. This is not to say that all herbs are entirely safe. Herbs such as foxglove must be treated with great care, and an overdose can be toxic. But, nevertheless, herbal remedies are gentler on our bodies than the potent chemical drugs prescribed by conventional medical practitioners.

The Holistic Approach

The holistic approach to treatment is vital to the understanding and practice of herbalism. Herbalists think that the danger of modern chemical drugs is due to the fact that the known active ingredient has been isolated and reproduced, usually at a potent level, whereas the known active ingredient in a herb is reinforced by many other substances, probably unrecognised, which are present in the plant and which can protect against harmful side-effects. For example, chemical diuretics are successful in their objective, which is to

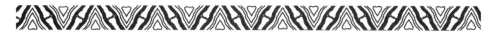

increase urine production. But their long-term use commonly causes potassium deficiency. Lack of potassium weakens nerves and muscle functions, lowers blood pressure and induces fatigue. Herbalists would prescribe dandelion as a diuretic: dandelion not only stimulates urine production but also contains large amounts of potassium, thus restoring any lost potassium and maintaining the body's stores of this mineral.

It is not just medicine which suffers from this 'isolationist' attitude. Sugar, for example, when still in raw cane form, contains a substance which actually guards against tooth decay. Food manufacturers, however, strip the cane of every ingredient and substance which it has leaving only the sucrose. The result, of course, is a very sweet substance, but one which decays teeth and is extremely fattening and even addictive.

Arguably, the 'isolationist' attitude includes the way in which our doctors are taught to heal. Presented with a patient who complains of, for example, recurring migraines, a remedy would be prescribed to stop the migraines occurring. A holistic practitioner, however, will want to know what type of migraine it is, what other symptoms may be present and the cause of the migraine. In other words, the holistic practitioner looks not just at the symptoms but at the whole state of health of the patient: not just at body parts and how they are functioning, but at emotional, mental and spiritual states. Holistic practitioners treat the whole person, not simply a part; they treat the individual, not the type. Holistic practitioners are consulted to maintain health, not simply to cure diseases; they regard good health as a positive, vital state, not just an absence of disease.

Herbs And Healing

To a herbal practitioner, the definition of a herb is much more general than it is to a chef. The leaves of plants are, of course, herbs, as are the roots. But also, the seeds are herbs, and the bark, and the flowers – in fact, all the anatomical parts of a plant which may be beneficial to healing and health come under the general description 'herb'. Furthermore, a herb is not restricted to a plant, but may be a moss, fungi or seaweed.

Nowadays, the equivalent of fast-food herbal preparations are available over the counter, usually in capsule form. But the genuine article can be conveniently taken in herbal teas, syrups, drops, inhaled or used in the form of ointment.

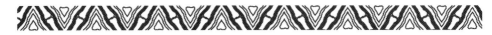

How Are The Herbs Effective?

Herbal formulae can be approximately described in one of three ways: as a means of eliminating and detoxifying accumulated poisons and harmful bacteria, as relaxants and tonics and as nourishment to the tissues, organs, blood and innate healing powers.

Herbal medicines are thought to trigger off neurochemical responses in the body which are a natural part of the healing process. By taking herbal medication in moderate doses over a period of time, these biochemical responses become automatic, even when the medication is discontinued.

Using Herbs

Since herbalism is holistic, it is employed to maintain overall good health. In this respect daily doses of garlic are beneficial for good circulation and for warding off infection. A herb such as chamomile is soothing and relaxing and can be enjoyed as a tea. Other ways of taking herbs in liquid form are as a decoction, infusion and tincture.

- *Decoction*: for preparations made from roots and bark. Put a heaped tablespoon of powdered dried herb into a stainless steel (not aluminium) saucepan, and pour in a pint of boiling water. Bring to the boil and allow to simmer for 10–15 minutes. Strain and drink.
- *Infusion*: fresh or dried herbs may be used in loose or tea bag form. The method is to warm a teapot and put in one dessertspoon of herb for each cup required. Pour in a cup of boiling water for each cup required and allow to steep for 10–15 minutes.
- *Tincture*: an alcohol-based concentrated preparation to be taken in small doses.

Herbs can be obtained from fresh food shops or may be found growing in the wild. If you decide to collect your own herbs, be sure that you know what you are picking, and harvest your herbs from an area which has not been sprayed with chemicals and which is not subject to the poisonous effects of car exhaust fumes. Pick only common herbs – nettle, for example, but not cowslip – and ensure that you are not harvesting a protected species.

An alternative may be to grow your own herbs: most herbs are hardy and are easily cultivated. You can obtain cuttings from your local garden centre, and some supermarkets now sell potted herbs. You can grow herbs indoors or in a window box.

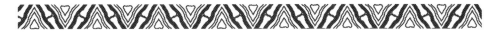

Western Herbalism

A professional medical herbalist is trained to carry out a full medical examination in much the same way as a GP, using the same type of equipment. Blood pressure, pulse reading, blood and urine samples may all be taken. Qualified medical herbalists are usually members of the National Institute of Medical Herbalists.

A medical herbalist can give more specialist advice on the use of herbal medicine for serious or long-term problems. Medical herbalists undergo a four-year course at the School of Herbal Medicine. At an initial consultation, a practitioner will ask the patient for details of his or her medical history, eating and exercise habits and whether stress is a factor in daily life. As a result of the overall diagnosis, the herbalist will prescribe a single herb or combination of herbs and specify in which form the medicine is to be taken, such as a tincture, as pills or as infusions.

Western Herbal Remedies For Arthritis And Rheumatism

The causes of arthritis and rheumatism may be due to any one or a combination of factors, including incorrect nutrition, bad posture, overexposure to cold and damp, a sluggish digestive system, hereditary factors, and so on. Herbal remedies will take account of the type of arthritis or rheumatism in order to treat it effectively. For example, a *rubefacient* herb may be applicable: this stimulates the blood circulation and can ease pain and local inflammation. Ginger and cayenne are rubefacient herbs and are rubbed into the local area for their benefit.

Diuretics help to eliminate toxins which may have caused the arthritis. Dandelion, yarrow and celery are all diuretics. Anti-inflammatories, such as meadowsweet, wild yam and black willow can reduce swellings and pain.

Blood purifiers cleanse the blood of toxins so that it can fulfil its normal nourishing role: celery is an effective blood purifier.

Valerian and chamomile are excellent relaxants and can help to relieve pain. They are also sedatives, which can be important if the pain is preventing sleep.

There are many, many herbs which are beneficial in relieving rheumatic or arthritic pain: far too many for one person to need at one time. Diagnosis from a professional herbalist is highly advisable. A herbalist will probably make up a special formula for you to treat

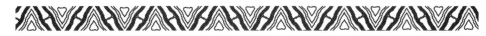

your particular type of pain, taking into account all the
requirements of your body.

Chinese Herbalism

Before prescribing any herbs, a Chinese herbalist will make a
thorough physical examination of which a large part is pulse
diagnosis. Using the index, middle and ring fingers on both wrists in
turn, the Chinese herbalist takes readings from each pulse which
together make up a composite diagnosis of each organ, limb and
circulatory state of health.

The healing philosophy of Chinese herbalism is founded on the
balance of *yin* and *yang*. *Yin* and *yang* are the opposite but
complementary aspects of everything in the natural world, including
humans, and their interrelationship. *Yin* qualities are dark, coldness
and inactivity; *yang* characteristics are light, heat and movement. If
yin dominates, the result is exhaustion, passivity, weakness; if *yang*
predominates, the result is irritability, excitability, hyperactivity. The
correct use of herbs can restore the balance of *yin* and *yang*.

According to Chinese principles, food is medicine and medicine
is food. Therefore a particular diet may be prescribed in
conjunction with a herbal remedy. In any case, Chinese food
contains many of the herbs used in medicine.

Chinese herbalists are usually found within the Chinese
communities, but you can obtain details of them from the Register
of Chinese Herbal Medicine (see page 63). Modern Chinese
herbalists tend to combine herbalism with acupuncture.

Chinese Herbal Remedies For Arthritis And Rheumatism

- *Zheng Gu Shui* is a tincture based on a Chinese folklore remedy. It has
  acquired worldwide recognition for its uses not only in relieving
  arthritic pains but also in relieving muscular pains generally. It is rubbed
  on to the troubled area and allowed to dry. It brings relief within hours.
- *I-Yi-Jen Tang* (*Coix lachryma-jobi*) is a herbal formula based on Job's Tears
  and six other herbs. It has also achieved wide recognition: the Japanese
  government approves its use in the treatment of arthritis. It is used for
  people who are in otherwise good health and who have a strong
  digestive system. It is available in capsule form, and is taken three times
  daily.

- *Shu-Ching-Huo-Hsieh-Tang* (clematis and stephania) is a herbal formula which contains 17 herbs. The Japanese government has also approved its use in the treatment of arthritis and related conditions. It is suitable for people whose health is weakened. The formula is available in capsule form and is taken three times daily.
- *Jenshen* (ginseng) has many uses, one of which is in the relief of arthritis and rheumatic pain. It can be taken in capsule or herbal tea forms to effect relief, again on a daily basis. However, it is best not to take it for more than 6–8 weeks without advice from a qualified herbal practitioner.
- *Han-Ch'In* (celery). Celery seeds are used to make a decoction and the tea taken two to three (or more) times daily. Sometimes a diet rich in celery is also prescribed.
- *Chinese Dragon Balm.* A herbal balm, the Dragon Balm relieves arthritic and rheumatic pain. It has also achieved worldwide recognition and is available from health food stores.

Dietary Considerations

In addition to using one of the above herbal remedies, both Chinese and Western herbalists may forbid fatty foods (such as pork and fried foods), white sugar and white flour products, bread and acidic fruit, and instead advocate plenty of celery and brown (unpolished) rice. Celery breaks down excessive acid and unpolished brown rice contains large amounts of the B vitamins.

Consulting A Herbalist

Western Medical Herbalists

For information, contact the National Institute of Medical Herbalists at 9 Palace Gate, Exeter EX1 1JA.

Chinese Herbalists

Traditional Chinese herbalists tend to be confined to Chinese centres, practising mainly within the Chinese community.

Contact the Register of Chinese Herbal Medicine at 138 Prestbury Road, Cheltenham GLS2 2DP.

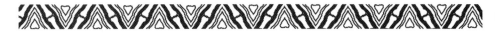

Ayurvedic And Unani Practitioners

Commonly known as Vaids and Hakims, these practitioners are mainly found within the Indian and Pakistani communities and offer treatment based on traditional principles.

Further Reading

A–Z of Modern Herbalism by Simon Mills (Diamond Books)
Herbal First Aid by Andrew Chevallier (Amberwood)
Herbalism: Headway Lifeguides by Francis Büning and Paul Hambly
    (Headway)
Herbal Medicine by Dian Dincin Buchman (Rider Books)
Secrets of the Chinese Herbalists by Richard Lucas (Lucas)
The New Holistic Herbal by David Hoffman (Element)
Traditional Home Herbal Remedies by Jan de Vries
    (Mainstream Publishing)

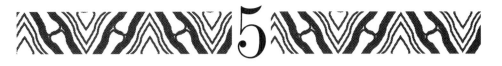

HOMOEOPATHY: VITAL JOINT FORCE

Homeopathy is based on the principle that 'Like cures like'. In other words, a substance which, in a healthy person, would bring about the symptoms of a particular disease can be used to treat a patient with that disease. The key to this is the homoeopathic understanding of symptoms and their role in disease and good health.

> 'Those who merely study and treat the effects of disease are like those who imagine that they can drive away winter by brushing snow from the door. It is not the snow that causes the winter but the winter that causes the snow.'

Paracelsus, who wrote those words, was a famous physician and philosopher of the fifteenth century. With these words he expressed a fundamental tenet of homoeopathy: that the symptoms are not the actual disease itself. Consequently, the strategy of suppressing the symptoms will not cure the disease. Furthermore, symptoms are an extremely important expression of the body's own healing abilities.

Conventional medicine treats symptoms as the disease itself and treatment is geared to suppressing the symptoms in order to cure an illness. Homoeopathy, on the other hand, encourages symptoms in order to speed the healing process. When the body falls prey to an infection, for example, influenza, it responds by producing the symptoms of a runny nose, watering eyes, fatigue, high temperature and so on. The runny nose, sneezing and watering eyes are all means by which the body is trying to expel the harmful agents. The fatigue forces the person to rest and thus allow the body to devote its energies to throwing off the 'flu. The high temperature is killing the harmful agents by literally burning them off.

The body is an extremely complex and sophisticated system and we are still discovering new things about it. Why should we doubt, then, that the body has its own methods of healing itself, of renewal and regeneration? And, having accepted that, should not we be helping our body to help itself? Taking a chemical cold remedy does the exact opposite: it overrides the body's natural functions and stops the symptoms of illness. Only when the body is unable to heal

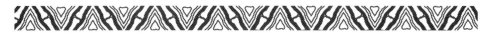

itself should intervention be necessary: unfortunately, orthodox drugs are not without their sometimes dangerous side-effects.

Two hundred years ago, a German doctor, Samuel Hahnemann (1755-1843), laid the foundations for modern homoeopathy. As a practising physician, he employed the then current techniques of blood letting, purges, leaching and administering strong enemas on patients, but he was at the same time aware that the fatality rate was much too high.

As a linguist, Hahnemann translated various medical texts. A text by the Scottish doctor Cullen espoused the healing abilities of cinchona bark in cases of malaria due, he thought, to cinchona bark's astringent qualities. Hahnemann was not convinced by this explanation of cinchona bark's efficacy: there were other astringent drugs and herbs available which did not alleviate malaria. His curiosity prompted him to dose himself with small amounts of cinchona bark over some days, and he was surprised to discover that he developed the symptoms of malaria himself. On ceasing the cinchona bark, the symptoms disappeared. This led him to the all-important conclusion that cinchona bark treats malaria because it produces the same symptoms as the disease itself. This in turn seemed to point to the conclusion that if you stimulate the symptoms of a disease, you can cure it; thus 'Like cures like'.

Hahnemann went on to experiment with other drugs both on himself and his followers. He called these experiments 'provings' and in this way laid the foundation of homoeopathic remedy pictures. He rejected allopathic medicine, seeing it as the antithesis of effective therapeutic treatment.

Homoeopathy developed, although not without opposition from orthodox medical practice. Many lives were saved during the European cholera epidemics by a homoeopathic remedy suggested by Hahnemann which used camphor. By the time of Hahnemann's death in 1843, homoeopathy was practised in most of Europe, Britain, Russia, South America and in the USA.

How Homoeopathy Works

Homoeopathy is based on three principles: the Law of Similars, the Single Remedy and the Minimal Dose:

- *The Law of Similars.* The human body, having its own extensive healing abilities, is encouraged to work through its own natural processes. In introducing a substance to the body which produces similar symptoms

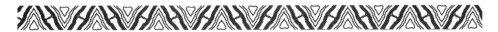

to the disease itself, the body is thereby stimulated in its own healing efforts. A correct homoeopathic prescription relies, therefore, on finding the most similar remedy to the disease state, as revealed through its symptoms.

- *The Single Dose.* Although the whole body is out of balance when an illness takes hold, only one remedy is given at a time. This allows the practitioner to study the effect the remedy has had before further prescriptions are made. Giving one remedy at a time is also a less confusing treatment for the body to deal with, as opposed to bombarding it with several factors which would dissipate its energies.
- *The Minimal Dose.* Because homoeopathy enhances present symptoms, only very small amounts of the remedies are necessary, since the body is already very sensitive. The specific potency and doses are prescribed by the homoeopath according to the individual patient's reaction to the disease and not according to the disease itself.

The concept of dilution is the greatest cause of scepticism from conventional practitioners: 'How can such minuscule amounts of an active ingredient benefit anybody?' they ask. Hahnemann did not know, and we are none the wiser today. Nevertheless, there is a great deal of empirical evidence that homoeopathy does succeed in treatment.

One of the many theories which seek to explain the success of homoeopathy turns away from a physical explanation and focuses instead on the holistic nature of the therapy. It may be that the potencies are acting at a very subtle level of energy and that these remedies vibrate or resonate with a person's 'vital force'. The right homoeopathic remedy is like a boost of subtle energy which returns the body to its proper frequency and so aids in recovery. Once the body is in tune, resonating at its proper rate, it is able to use its immune system to throw off the toxins that cause illness.

Whatever the explanation, the fact remains that homoeopathy is effective. Because of this, there are five National Health homoeopathic hospitals in Britain; clinical trials have substantiated homoeopathy's validity and, worldwide, homoeopathy is a flourishing therapy.

Hering's Laws Of Cure

Constantin Hering was a German practitioner who emigrated to America in the 1830s. He was already a firm espouser of

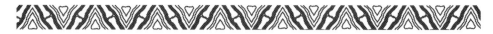

homoeopathy and he introduced it to his new country. He established three principles to describe the healing process when homoeopathy is applied.

First, Hering observed that healing operates from within and works its way outwards according to the depth of the symptoms. He described the layers of healing, commencing with the most fundamental and ending with the least serious: the brain, the heart, the liver, the bones, the muscles and finally the skin. Assuming that the skin is a problem, and that the condition appeared chronologically after a liver disorder, for example, it may be that while the liver responds well to treatment, the skin may worsen as the toxins are eliminated. If, on the other hand, the skin improves when it is the liver which is the problem, the homoeopath knows he or she has not prescribed the correct remedy.

The second of Hering's laws of cure states that symptoms reappear and disappear in their reverse chronological order of appearance: heart disease, for example, is the end result of a gradual accumulation of standard symptoms. To cure heart disease the contributory factors must first be dealt with, such as lifestyle, diet, work habits etc. Homoeopaths have observed recurrences of past illnesses which have led to the current illness.

The third of Hering's laws of cure states that healing moves from the upper to the lower parts of the body, in stages. For example, rheumatic stiffness in the shoulder which heals but is replaced by stiffness in the hip is considered to a positive sign of progressive healing.

Homoeopathic practitioners have found that Hering's laws are sometimes in reverse: that healing is effected from the lower body to the upper, or that the outer responds before the inner. In such cases the patient's overall sense of improvement is vital to continued prescriptions and treatment.

Homoeopathic Medicines

Many substances have been found to be effective for homoeopathic treatment. Not only plants, but also minerals, chemical compounds and bacterial extracts are used in homoeopathic medicines. Since the aim is to enhance the symptoms of a disease, it is perhaps not surprising that even poisons, such as arsenic, mercury, snake venom and deadly nightshade, are employed. Today there are over 2,500 medicines available.

The medicines are made up by taking the raw material through a process of serial dilution and vigorous shaking, called *succussion*. Each stage of succussion increases the potency, or strength, which is given a number and a letter. Potencies with an 'X' affix are diluted1:9 and those with a 'C' affix are diluted 1:99 at each successive stage. Plant materials are instantly soluble, but minerals and metals need to undergo a process called *trituration* (grinding) with a milk/sugar powder up to the 3X potency before they become soluble; at that point the dilution and succussion process continues in the same manner as plants.

Homoeopathic medicines are widely available from pharmacies and health food stores. Although the lower potencies of 6C or 30C are generally available packaged for over-the-counter sale, caution is advised in the repetiton of the 30C, as this is a relatively high potency. There are creams, ointments and lotions for external use.

A Visit To A Homoeopath

A homoeopath may be a conventionally trained doctor who has gone on to study homoeopathy, in which case you may receive a full medical check up to include blood pressure tests and so on, or may only have trained in homoeopathy. The homoeopathic consultation really starts with the many questions which will be asked of you. Beginning with your immediate health concern, close questioning of the type of symptoms you experience will be vital in prescribing the correct remedy. Next, establishing a picture of you and your type of lifestyle will be important: are you constantly on the go, or do you lead a sedentary life? Do you sleep well at nights and for how long? Do you feel the cold unduly? What are your preferred foods? The questioning attempts to establish your emotional, mental and spiritual state. Homoeopathy, as a holistic therapy, treats the whole individual on all levels and does not treat an isolated part.

Homoeopathy And Relief For Arthritis And Rheumatism Sufferers

In 1980 a double-blind trial ('Homoeopathic Therapy in Rheumatoid Arthritis: Evaluation by Double-Blind Trial', R G Gibson, S L M Gibson, A D MacNeil, et al.) was carried out to investigate the efficacy of homoeopathic remedies in sufferers of

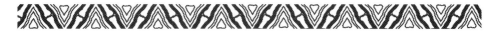

RA. Each volunteer was prescribed an individual homoeopathic remedy but only half were given the actual treatment, while the other half were given a placebo (an inactive substance). Eighty-two per cent of those given the homoeopathic remedies showed an improvement, but only 21 per cent of the placebo takers experienced the same degree of improvement.

This study highlights two important factors about arthritis and homoeopathy. The first is that homoeopathy does relieve arthritic pain. The second is that each volunteer was prescribed his or her individual remedy. It is not possible to list here a definitive cure for arthritis or rheumatism because homoeopathy is based on an individual prescription, and because chronic diseases do need the attention of a qualified practitioner.

When arthritis or rheumatism might be hereditary, it is obviously particularly important that appropriate steps are taken to prevent the onset of the disease; if you are in current good health, preventative measures are better than looking for a cure later.

Stress has a lot to answer for. One of the consequences of stress is that calcium is withdrawn from the skeleton to mitigate its effects. If this happens frequently, the body's stores of calcium will be depleted, perhaps to the extent of weakening the skeleton itself. If blood levels of calcium stay high and are not reduced to their normal level, calcium deposits collect in the muscles and/or joints.

Alternatively, overproduction of uric acid collects in the joints and/or muscles. In this case, the diet is altered to avoid acid-producing foods. Homoeopathic medicines can speed the expellation of accumulated acid and return the balance to normal.

In Conversation With A Practitioner

Q. How long does treatment take?
A. This is a difficult question to answer, but after several interviews the homoeopath is better able to give you an idea of this. The nature of your complaint, its severity and how long you have been suffering from it, will all influence your body's ability to respond to treatment. Remember that arthritis and rheumatism in particular are chronic diseases which have taken a long time to develop: a quick cure is not, therefore, a realistic expectation.

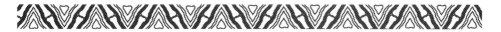

Q. How many appointments are necessary?
A. During the first six months visits may be frequent but will taper off as you become healthier. We feel we need to see you initially more frequently (follow-ups are usually every four to six weeks in the beginning) to work with you and evaluate your progress. Yet we are not insensitive to the cost of treatment and do not wish to make this a burden. A happy medium can be reached.

If a remedy has brought your system into balance, in our experience this state can last for a long time. We would then need to wait until the next 'remedy picture' comes up clearly. This is the time to have renewed faith in your body's healing abilities.

Q. How can I be involved?
A. You don't have to believe in homoeopathic remedies in order for them to work (we treat babies and there are homoeopathic vets). But to select the correct remedy and for the treatment to continue to act, your co-operation and commitment are necessary.
You can help by:

- Noting any changes after you take the remedy – keeping a weekly journal can be helpful for bringing to your follow-up consultations. Please note general changes as well as specific ones.
- Giving a clear and complete account of your symptoms on all levels.
- Above all, communicating any concerns or questions you may have. We are always trying to find better ways of helping you and welcome your comments.

Q. Where do I obtain my remedies?
A. We either have your remedy available at the clinic and will dispense it, the cost usually being included in your consultation fee, or we shall refer you to a convenient homoeopathic pharmacy.

Although there are over 2,000 remedies which are prepared in established homoeopathic pharmacies, most homoeopathic prescriptions are made from a narrower range of 200–300 remedies.

Q. Can homoeopathic treatment be undertaken at the same time as other alternative therapies, for example, acupuncture and chiropractic?
A. Following the principle of the single dose, we advise against other types of treatment while you are taking homoeopathic remedies. This is because we need to establish which remedies are successful and which are not: if you are receiving acupuncture at the same time, a homoeopathic practitioner will not know if it is his/her prescription which is resulting in any changes, or if it is due to the acupuncture. An acupuncturist would also prefer that you follow one type of therapy at a time. Similarly,

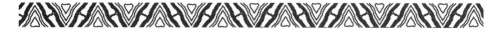

essential oils can interfere with homoeopathy and should preferably be avoided while following a homoeopathic prescription.

Concerning chiropractic and osteopathy and their treatment while undergoing homeopathic treatment, we have found that mild manipulative therapy does not interfere with homoeopathy.

Q. Can a wrong remedy be given and what are the effects?
A. As much as we carefully try to match the correct remedy, we do not always achieve 100 per cent accuracy. If appropriately used, homoeopathic treatment should produce no side-effects from the remedies. Either nothing changes or the true symptom picture will become even clearer and the right remedy is more obvious.

It can take several interviews for a homoeopath to get an accurate picture of the totality of your symptoms and an 'essential' understanding of this to select the right remedy. Of course, the clearer and more in touch you are with yourself the easier this task becomes.

Q. What about seeing a GP?
A. Homoeopathy is complementary to the health care that is available. We recommend you maintain your relationship with your doctor, especially for routine needs and emergencies. Your GP will also arrange for you to have any blood tests, X-rays, etc, or refer you to a consultant.

Finding A Practitioner

An increasing number of qualified medical doctors now offer homoeopathic treatment. Most of them have taken a postgraduate training course to become a Member or a Fellow of the Faculty of Homoeopathy (MFHom or FFHom). A register of practitioners is maintained by the Faculty of Homoeopathy, c/o the Royal London Homoeopathic Hospital, Great Ormond Street, London WC1N 3HR. Many of the professional homoeopaths have trained for four years at accredited colleges and have become graduate or registered members of the Society of Homoeopaths (RSHom). For a list of registered homoeopaths, write to The Society of Homoeopaths, 2 Artizan Road, Northampton NN1 4HU.

In addition to the private and NHS practitioners there are five NHS homoeopathic hospitals, in London, Bristol, Tunbridge Wells, Liverpool and Glasgow. There are also a number of private clinics nationally. Further information may be obtained from The British Homoeopathic Association, 27A Devonshire Street, London W1N 1RJ.

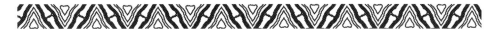

Further Reading

Everybody's Guide to Homoeopathic Medicines by Stephen Cummings
and Dana Ullman (Gollancz)

Homoeopathy For Babies and Children by Beth MacEoin (Headway)

Homoeopathy for Emergencies by Phyllis Speight (C W Daniels)

Homoeopathy: Headway Lifeguides by Beth MacEoin (Headway)

Homoeopathy, Medicine for the New Man by George Vithoulkas
(Thorsons)

Homoeopathy: Medicine for the 21st Century by Dana Ullman
(Thorsons)

The Complete Homoeopathy Handbook: A Guide to Everyday Health Care
by Miranda Castro (Macmillan)

*The Family Guide to Homoeopathy: The Safe Form of Medicine for the
Future* by Andrew Lockie (Elm Tree Books)

ANTHROPOSOPHICAL MEDICINE: ORGANISATION OF BODY WARMTH

Orthodox medicine is based upon hypothesis and experimentation; if something cannot be proven by experiment, it does not exist as a scientific fact. This premise can lead to an oversimplification, if it is applied to the physical aspect of existence only. Indeed, in conventional medicine (based on natural science) this simplification is a fundamental tenet, and we call it *reductionism*. All aspects of our existence – the physical, the manifestations of living organisms, the emotional and mental or spiritual aspects – are reduced to mere expressions of the physical.

In anthroposophical medicine, the methods and discipline of (natural) science are applied to other, non-physical levels of reality. Anthroposophy is also called a spiritual science; it acknowledges the other levels of our existence and investigates their inter-relationships. This approach broadens the possibilities of treatment of illness.

Anthroposophy was founded by the Austrian philosopher and scientist Rudolf Steiner (1861–1925); he outlined the philosophical foundations of his ideas in his treatise *The Philosophy of Freedom*. Steiner describes in this, and other works, how the human being has not just a body, but also a soul and spirit. He discerns four aspects to the bodily nature of the human being; health and well-being depends on a harmonious working together of these aspects.

Together with a Dutch doctor, Ita Wegman, Steiner further developed his ideas for medicine, and they wrote the book which marked the beginning of anthroposophical medicine: *The Fundamentals of Therapy*.

The Four Aspects Of The Human Being

In addition to the physical body, three other elements are present in the human body which complete the picture of the human being. In anthroposophical terms they are called the *etheric* (or life-)body, the *astral* (or sentient-) body and the *ego* (-body). These elements are

common to us all, but cannot be perceived directly by the ordinary physical senses. Essentially the *etheric* body is concerned with growth, repair and replenishment, the *astral* body represents the sentient and emotional life, and the *ego* embodies the individual spiritual core, which man alone possesses.

The Etheric Body

This is the force which governs the existence of the physical body. It imbues the physical body with life, without which the physical body deteriorates and disintegrates; this happens naturally after death, when only physical laws govern. The etheric body is responsible for keeping the physical parts of the body into a whole and maintaining its integrity by continuous repair and restructuring. It is the very source of our natural tendency to heal and recover from less serious ailments, without additional medical help. In short, the etheric body constantly guards against death and decay (physical laws).

The Anthroposophical Elements Of A Complete Person			
Spirit	Self-consciousness	Human	Ego
Soul	Consciousness	Animal	Astral body
Life	Life	Plant	Etheric body
Material	Weighable and measurable	Mineral	Physical body

The Astral Body

The astral body represents the soul element, common to animals and humans, and differentiates them from the plants and minerals. Our sentient being, consciousness as such, is carried by the astral body.

It is through our sentient (astral) body, that we are aware of emotions, feelings, thoughts: a level which cannot be measured tangibly, but is very much a reality. A conventional doctor believes that this aspect of our existence is a mere manifestation of physical and chemical processes. An anthroposophical practitioner regards the sentient life and therefore the sentient (or astral) body as a reality, just as much as the physical.

The astral body has, generally speaking, a strong *catabolic* (breaking down) effect in the human body, and so has an opposite effect to the etheric body, which is constantly endeavouring to build

and repair. So, good health prevails for as long as the destructive (*catabolic*) processes, due to the activity of the astral body, are held in check and in equilibrium by the building (*anabolic*) activity of the etheric body. An imbalance between the two will result in illness.

The Ego

Present only in the human being, the ego adds an additional level of consciousness, namely the self-consciousness. It comprises the ability to think independently and brings an awareness of being autonomous. So humans are able to refrain from instinctive behaviour, if reasoning leads them: a quality that is not present in the animal world. The human ability to learn, develop and become an independent and lonely being, is due to the ego, the spiritual core of man. On a bodily level, this ego has quite a complicated task and influences, generally speaking, the etheric body in an anabolic way and joins the astral body in its catabolic activity. However, the ego always guards the totality of the bodily processes and works mainly through the warmth organisation of the body.

The Anthroposophical View of Illness

Anthroposophical practitioners look at health and illness in terms of the interrelationships between the ego, the astral body, the etheric body and the physical body. These four aspects of the human being interrelate and interconnect to each other in different parts of the body and its organ systems.

The three main functional organ systems within anthroposophical medical thought are described as the nerve–sense system, the metabolic limb system and the rhythmical system.

The nerve–sense system comprises, physically, the central nervous system (brain, sense organs, spinal cord) and the whole of the autonomous nervous system (connecting to all the internal organs).

This organ system lacks vitality, regeneration and movement. The nervous system is very vulnerable and easily damaged if deprived of oxygen and other nutrients. The life-bringing activity of the etheric body is therefore very minimal, and the catabolic action of the astral body dominates, bringing about consciousness, thought and perception.

In the metabolic limb system we find a wealth of vital activity in the main digestive organs (liver, pancreas, stomach etc.), the

lymphatic system and our reproductive organs. The muscles of our limbs are the main consumers of nutrients and are full of life and movement.

There is no consciousness in this system and we are not aware of its anabolic processes, unless there is something wrong and we feel pain; pain is heightened consciousness, and is experienced through our astral or sentient body. The astral body also works in the metabolic limb system, but here not in a catabolic way. It serves the predominantly anabolic activity of the etheric body. Whilst in the nerve–sense system the catabolic activity overrules the anabolic.

The tension between the catabolic and anabolic processes in these two organ systems is regulated by a third functional activity–that of the rhythmical system.

The Three Systems In Anthroposophical Medicine

Nerve–Sense:	Thinking	Conscious	Cooling Catabolic Hardening
Rhythmic:	Feeling	Dream-like	Balancing Mediating
Metabolic Limb:	Volition	Unconscious	Warming Anabolic Softening

This rhythmical system of the body is found most clearly in the rhythmical activity of the heart, circulation and breathing: *systole* (contraction) and *diastole* (expansion), in-breath and out-breathing, illustrate the constantly changing balance of the rhythmical system. It incorporates and balances both the primarily catabolic action of the nerve–sense system (contraction, consciousness enhancing), and the mainly anabolic activity of the metabolic limb system (relaxation, regeneration).

Such a dynamic and artistic view of the functions of the human body enables the anthroposophical doctor to relate anatomical and physiological aspects to psychological and spiritual aspects in the human being. Illness and dis-ease result from imbalances in the interrelating systems. Such an understanding broadens the scope of diagnosis as well as treatment. Different methods of treatment are used to achieve this.

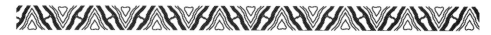

The Medicines

When and where appropriate and/or necessary, conventional medicines are and will be used. However, the remedies developed in anthroposophical medicine are derived from plant or mineral and, occasionally, animal sources. The choice of substance is based on the perceived relationship between the life process in the human body and nature. Steiner gave many indications of how certain substances relate to bodily processes and organs; for example, he indicated how the seven metals (lead, tin, iron, copper, mercury, silver and gold) correspond to organs and organ-processes. So an anthroposophical practitioner might prescribe a potentised preparation of tin, as drops or in the form of an ointment, for a patient with liver problems, or copper for regulation of the kidney function. Plant substances may well be given in material doses, as well as in potentised form.

Artistic Therapies

Artistic activity engages and appeals to the creative sources of the human being; the aim in therapy would be to mobilise such creative potential, and not particularly to create a work of art as such. Being engaged in a creative process also influences our bodily functions, in different and often subtle ways. Painting with a blue colour only will have a calming effect on our breathing and circulation, whilst sculpture work will engage our will more directly. For both physiological and psychological reasons, activities such as music, painting, form-drawing and sculpture may be recommended as part of an integral treatment plan.

Eurythmy Therapy

This therapy developed out of the art-form *eurythmy*, which Steiner also called *visible speech* or *visible music*. It is an art of movement (dance) through which the formative and creative forces of the world are made visible, in an artistic way. The eurythmy therapist uses specific gestures that express, for instance, certain vowels or consonants in a certain sequence. Through these movements, a soul-mood is created and they engender changes in the breathing, circulation and distribution of muscular tension. The exercises are used in the treatment of both physical and psychological disorders.

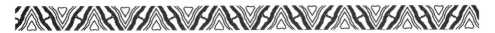

Hydrotherapy And Massage

In these treatments, the physical body is more directly addressed. A special form of rhythmical massage was developed, which in comparison with other forms of massage, is quite gentle. The masseur will identify patterns of muscular tension, warmth penetration and distribution, and the tone of the skin and underlying soft tissues. Particularly the irregularities of the warmth organisation are noted, as the warmth as such is regarded as the physical medium through which the activity of the ego works. Through addressing the warmth, with oil-dispersion baths and using particular aromatic oils in the massage itself, a self-sustaining improvement and redistribution of warmth and tension can be achieved. Particularly the rhythmical system is strengthened in relation to the other functional systems; the breathing relaxes and deepens, a healthier flow of warmth comes about, relieving inappropriate tensions.

The Treatment Of Rheumatism and Arthritis

These are degenerative and deforming conditions of the joints. The bony surfaces of the joints are progressively destroyed, and active inflammation is present. Generally speaking, inflammation and fever are regarded as part of a healthy bodily response to invasion (bacteria or other micro-organisms) and internal deformities (as in cancer, for instance). In fever/inflammation, the ego activity engages the astral activity and strongly guides it into an anabolic direction. Feverish illnesses follow a specific pattern and are usually self-limiting. The immune system is strengthened with every invasion of the body that is successfully dealt with. When there exists an underlying anabolic (ether) weakness, and the catabolic (destructive) activity of the astral body starts to dominate, localised destructive inflammatory problems arise; the warmth organisation loses its grip and is unable to intervene. In degenerative joint disease, this problem results in increasing rigidity and deformities. It follows that the primary aim of therapy must be to strengthen both the warmth organisation and the etheric (anabolic) activity. In an active (inflammatory) phase of joint disease, any treatment should be carefully monitored because of the risk of the condition flaring up. Medicines, rest and dietary measures would be the main brunt of anthroposophical treatment then. In the more quiescent phase of

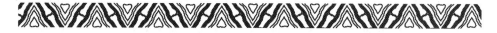

illness, more challenging treatments can be introduced. With pyrogenic and/or sulphur baths, the disturbed warmth activity is addressed; through the pyrogenic bath, the body temperature is carefully increased and the body is 'pushed' into a better distribution of warmth and learns to maintain it after repeated treatments.

Eurythmy therapy and painting therapy will usually be added at some stage of the treatment.

Finding A Practitioner

Anthroposophical practitioners are all qualified medical doctors who have taken a further postgraduate course recognised by the Anthroposophical Medical Association in Britain. Some may be found working in the NHS, although others work privately or in the Rudolf Steiner schools and homes for children in need of special care (Camphill Communities). Residential treatment is also available.

Consultations are very much like seeing a GP except that there may be additional details and questions about, for example, lifestyle and emotional situation. Diagnosis is made in the same way as a GP and treatment is prescribed depending on the individual characteristics of the patient.

Treatment will range from conventional, anthroposophical or herbal to homoeopathic types of medication. In addition, eurythmy, massage, hydrotherapy or an art therapy may be prescribed to complement and enhance the treatment.

The Anthroposophical Medical Association maintains a register of members. It is based at the Park Attwood Therapeutic Centre, Trimpley, Bewdley, Worcestershire DY12 1RE.

Further Reading

Anthroposophical Medicine by Dr M Evans and I Rodger (Thorsons)
Anthroposophical Medicine and its Remedies by Otto Wolf (Weleda Ag)
Rudolf Steiner: Scientist of the Invisible by A P Shepherd (Floris Books)

ACUPUNCTURE, ACUPRESSURE AND REFLEXOLOGY: POWERFUL POINTS

Acupuncture, acupressure and reflexology are all based on the essentials of Chinese philosophy which state that all living mater is activated by a life force, or energy, called *chi*. The *chi* flows in the human body along channels which are called *meridians*. As long as the channels of energy are kept open, unhindered by blockages, the *chi* can flow freely and with it optimum health is maintained.

The free flow of *chi* is disturbed when two opposing but complementary aspects, *yin* and *yang*, are out of balance. *Yin* characteristics are female, darkness, inactivity, wet and cold. *Yang* characteristics are male, light, movement, dryness and heat. Harmony only exists when *yin* and *yang* are in perfect balance. Treatment is based on restoring the balance of *yin* and *yang*, which restores the free flow of *chi*. One of the best-known methods of achieving this balance is acupuncture, in which the body's energy network is entered by inserting needles to stimulate specific points. Another is to stimulate the points by way of finger pressure and massage; this is called acupressure. Yet another is to stimulate points on the feet using finger pressure; this is called reflexology.

For the purposes of acupuncture and acupressure, classically there were 365 points, now there are more than 1,000 points on the body which lie on 12 meridians. Ten of the meridians are named after certain organs to which they relate, that is, the large intestine, stomach, heart, spleen, small intestine, bladder, kidney, gall bladder, lung and liver.

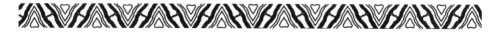

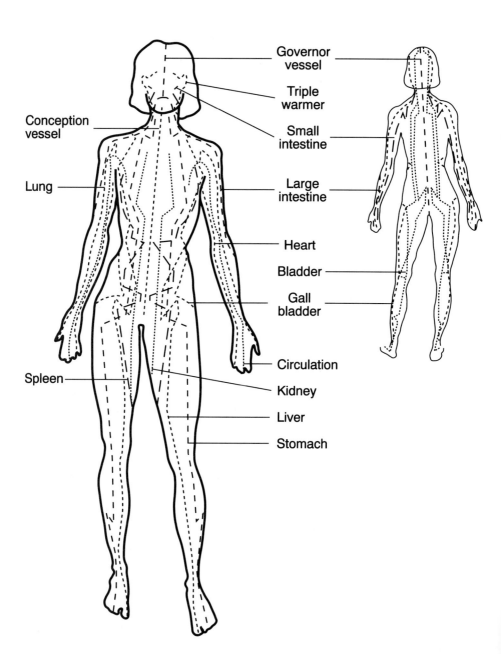

The meridians

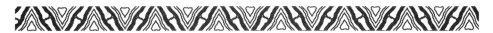

Acupuncture

Acupuncture is now widely practised in the West, and the modern Western School of acupuncture is frequently used in NHS pain clinics.

How Does Acupuncture Work?

Sceptics attribute the success of acupuncture to the patient's desire for it to work. This theory however is disproved each time an 'unbeliever' tries the therapy, and is surprised to find that it has helped to restore health.

Acupuncture was first promoted in the West by the American commentator, James Reston, who visited Peking in the 1970s. While there he suffered acute appendicitis. This was successfully operated on using a local anaesthetic, but his post-operative pain was treated with acupuncture. This impressed him so much that he and his wife visited other parts of China and on his return to the USA, he did much to focus both professional and public attention on this therapy.

One theory as to the success of acupuncture is that its practice stimulates the body to release its natural painkillers, the *endorphins* and *enkephalins*. These natural hormones must be present to avoid or resist depression. Another notion is that of the 'gate control' theory: this states that there are neuropathway 'gates' to the brain via the spinal chord. Anaesthetic acupuncture is believed to 'close the gates', blocking the pain messages so that we do not feel the pain.

However, these theories do not account for the success of acupuncture in the treatment of skin conditions, an inability to sleep at night, high blood pressure and a host of other complaints.

Diagnosis

The acupuncturist will take a full medical history, and note the condition of the patient's skin, hair, eyes, tongue, body odour, voice tone and so on. Some acupuncturists also take readings of the patient's blood pressure and weight in the manner of a GP, but this is not part of traditional Chinese practice.

Pulse diagnosis is an extremely skilled and complex matter which takes years to master and increasingly is not used by modern acupuncturists who do not subscribe to its use. The traditional

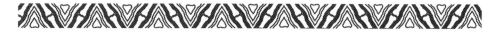

acupuncturist, however, places the index, middle and ring finger of his right hand on the patient's left wrist and takes six readings which are described in one of 28 terms including 'weak', 'thin', 'light', 'tight', 'fine', 'hasty' and then does the same for the opposite wrist using his left hand. This exhaustive pulse diagnosis gives the practitioner an insight into the health of the person's individual organs, circulatory and immune systems and much more, and forms the basis of the prescription.

Using Needles

This is the part of the treatment which makes the potential patient feel queasy, but it is not a painful sensation – the needles only produce a slight tingling sensation – and, when carried out correctly, no blood is drawn.

The needles are made of stainless steel and are very fine. They are inserted just below the skin, vertically, obliquely or almost horizontally. The needles are left in for a varying length of time, from a few minutes to 45 minutes, and during this time they are manipulated, that is, rotated to stimulate the meridian. Sometimes deeper penetration is called for, to a depth of $\frac{1}{2}$ to $1\frac{1}{4}$ inches, but again this is not painful.

A technique known as *moxibustion* is sometimes employed to stimulate further the meridians. A ball of mugwort herb is placed on the needle's handle and set alight. A gentle heat travels down the needle and into the body.

Acupuncture points are associated with decreased electrical impulses, and can be identified by passing electrical charges down a needle into the skin.

A modern form of acupuncture uses electrical pulses which are passed down a needle-like device which is not in fact inserted under the skin. This is used as an occasional, useful adjunct to acupuncture.

Auriculotherapy

The ear is said to resemble the human foetus with its head pointing downwards. As a result, a correlation has been established between points on the ear and the rest of the body. Many acupuncture prescriptions include stimulation of the ear as well as the main body itself. Usually an electronic instrument is used to detect the low

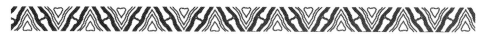

energy points and to stimulate them; however, needles are
sometimes used.

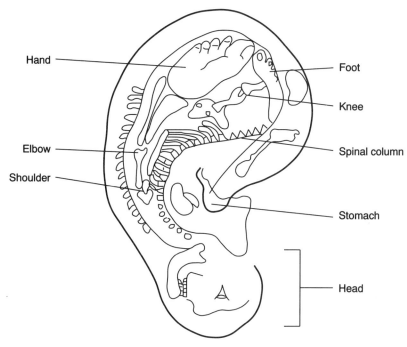

The human body reflected in the ear

The number of needles used can vary. Usually the higher the skill
of the acupuncturist, the fewer are the needles used. The type of
treatment required will also have a bearing on the number used.

After the needles are removed, a general sense of relaxation
follows.

Acupuncture And Arthritis And Rheumatism

The undisputed efficacy of acupuncture as a pain relief has made it
a popular choice for sufferers of arthritis and rheumatism. Arthritic
pain in the hip would target the meridians which, perhaps
surprisingly, affects the gall bladder (GB 34, 30, 29) and the liver
(Liv 6, 11). Auricular points which may be stimulated could include
the buttock point, gall bladder and bladder (B 11).

Arthritis in the knee would additionally need stimulation of the
Governor Vessel (GV 3) and stomach meridians (St 37, 38). Arthritis
in the ankle would be treated differently according to whether the
foot is turned inwards or outwards.

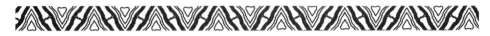

A regular course of treatment may be necessary while attention is also paid to diet in an attempt to either halt the progress of onset of arthritis or, if it is chronic, to provide some relief from the pain.

Acupressure

When you hold your forehead or press your temples when you have a headache you are instinctively using acupressure to relieve the pain. The Chinese discovered more than 5,000 years ago that applying pressure to certain points on the body brings relief from pain. The Japanese name for the therapy is *Shiatsu*.

When pressure is applied to certain points on the body it stimulates the flow of blood: this can relieve muscular and emotional tension and encourages the body's own healing systems to come into force.

The points used are the same as in acupuncture, but while acupuncture has been the target of much scientific research, acupressure (the older of the two therapies) has been largely overlooked. However, acupressure is enjoying increasing popularity because it requires no special instruments – just your fingers and hands. It can be practised at any time and anywhere.

How It Works

Tension and stress tend to accumulate around the *potent points* of the body, as they are called. The Chinese believe that *chi* passes through the potent points. Keeping the potent points open allows the *chi* to flow freely. It also elongates the muscle fibres and stimulates the blood flow and lymphatic circulation, so the overall immune system benefits.

Stimulation of the potent points also releases endorphins. When endorphins are released, not only is pain sensitivity blocked but oxygen flow increases; this enables the muscles to relax.

There are three types of potent points: local, trigger and tonic.

- *Local point.* This is the area where pain or discomfort is felt. Application to the local point will bring relief.
- *Trigger point.* This triggers a reflex in another part of the body. The triggering mechanism is believed to be effective because the stimulus is carried through the meridians.
- *Tonic points.* These are points which effect maintenance of good health. A popular tonic point is in the webbing between the thumb and the index finger.

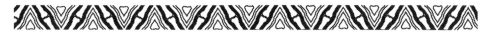

As with the meridians, the names of the potent points offers an insight into their use. For example, Shoulder Corner benefits the shoulder, Three Mile Point is said to give enough energy to run three miles, and Lung Associated Point benefits lung disorders. Additionally, each point has a classification number which is used by acupressurists and acupuncturists alike.

Practising Acupressure

There are four main ways of applying pressure: firmly, slowly, brisk rubbing and quick tapping. For general toning and improving the circulation, pressure is just applied for a few seconds. However, if there is actual pain or discomfort, the pressure would be held longer, for several minutes. Slow, kneading movements will relax stiff muscles, and a brisk rubbing action will not only improve circulation but stop chills and numbness. For the delicate facial area, quick tapping using just the fingertips improves circulation and nerve functioning.

Ideally, you should practise acupressure on a daily basis, for an hour at the most, but two or three times a week will also net benefits.

Potent Points For Arthritis And Rheumatism

The following will be of interest to sufferers:

- *Joining the Valley (LI 4)* relieves arthritic pain in the hands, shoulder, neck and elbow. It is found in the webbing between the thumb and first finger. Simply press this point using your thumb and index finger, gradually applying pressure to the bone underneath the index finger. Hold for a couple of minutes and then do the same to the other hand. *(Caution: pregnant women should not use this point because it can cause premature contraction of the uterus.)*
- *Outer Gate (TW5)* is on the outer part of your forearm, 2 ½ finger widths up from the wrist crease. Use the knuckles to apply firm pressure for a couple of minutes, and do the same to the other hand.
- *Three Mile Point (St 36)*. To find this measure 4 finger widths down from your kneecap, and a half inch outwards from the shinbone. Move your foot up and down; the muscle should be felt. Using your fist, apply pressure to massage up and down both legs, for about a minute. This benefits the whole body.
- *Gates of Consciousness (GB 20)*. This is found at the base of the skull, at the back, in the hollows which are about 2–3 inches apart. Press these

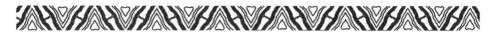

indentations with your thumbs and slowly tilt back your head as you do so. Hold for 1 minute and gently ease off the pressure and allow your head to slowly come forward. This potent point not only relieves an arthritic neck, or shoulders, but is useful for general relaxation and easing tension and migraines.

There are many other potent points which may be beneficial to sufferers. A professional acupressure massage would give you the opportunity to experience the full benefits, and teach you how to administer the technique yourself.

Acupressure Massage

There are several massage techniques and each therapist has his or her own way of working. Practitioners will usually use a firm thumb or the fingertips to massage the pain relieving points, although some may use palms, elbows and even knees.

The sessions may last between 30 to 60 minutes. Depending on your condition, they may be needed for several weeks or longer.

Since acupressure lends itself to self-administration, it is not vital to visit a practitioner. However, a course in the technique would net better results than teaching yourself from a book.

Reflexology

Reflexology connects certain points on the feet with the rest of the body. Unlike auricular acupuncture, which is an additional technique used by acupuncturists, reflexology is a therapy in its own right.

Although an American doctor, Dr Fitzgerald, drew up the chart of reflexology as it is used today, the Ancient Egyptians and Chinese first discovered the link between the feet and the rest of the body thousands of years ago. Drawings on ancient Egyptian tombs show massage being applied to the feet, while traditional Chinese medicine has always applied massage to the feet to affect the organs of the body.

Modern reflexology owes much to Dr Fitzgerald's description of 'zone therapy'. He discovered that operations on the throat and nose caused a great deal of discomfort to some of his patients but not to others. Further investigation showed that those patients who had escaped the pain had applied pressure to parts of their hands quite unconsciously.

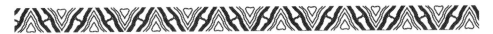

Dr Fitzgerald began his investigations in 1913. He divided the body up into ten longitudinal zones, from the head down to the toes and out through the fingers. He believed that the body's bioelectrical energy flowed down these pathways to various reflex points in the hands and feet. A few doctors received his comments seriously, and in particular Eunice Ingham developed the technique of reflexology which concentrated on the soles and tops of the feet, and the toes. Reflexology was introduced into Britain by a protégée of Ingham, Doreen Bayly.

As time went on, a link was made between reflexology and acupuncture, although Dr Fitzgerald saw the two therapies as quite distinct; he believed that reflexology was successful because it affected the six major meridians which run through the feet.

The Link Between The Feet And The Body

A reflexology chart will show the parts of the body drawn on to the feet. The left foot corresponds with the left side of the body and the right foot with the right side of the body. The big toes represent the head and brain, the little toes the sinuses and the area just below the toes represents the eyes and ears. The knees and pelvic regions are situated towards the heels.

The principle of reflexology's active effects is based on the channels of energy which run throughout the body and which reach the reflex parts of the feet. Obstruction of the energy causes blockages which can be felt by an experienced reflexologist as minute deposits in the feet. The reflexologist manipulates the area to dissolve the physical blockage which, once effected, releases the blocked meridian.

As well as dissolving deposits, reflexology can be used to dilate blood vessels and stimulate or sedate certain areas of the body. It is thought that endorphins can also be released as a result of massaging the feet. Endorphins are produced by the pituitary gland and stop the passage of pain signals through the spinal nerves. The brain reacts to pain by sending a message to the pituitary gland that more endorphins should be produced, until the system is overloaded and the number of messages which can reach the brain is limited.

Uses Of Reflexology

Reflexology is used to alleviate simple everyday ailments, such as colds, headaches and sore throats. Chronic diseases require treatment by a doctor.

Its other, perhaps more important, use, is as a diagnostic tool. If a blockage is felt in a particular part of the foot, its corresponding organ will be identified as a troublespot. However, the severity and type of illness cannot be identified from reflexology.

Reflexology has a place as a preventative therapy: by keeping the body's overall functions in good order, and by acting as an early warning system of potential illness.

A Visit To A Reflexologist

A reflexologist will begin by enquiring into your general state of health and asking about your lifestyle, the amount of exercise you take, type of diet which you enjoy, and the level of stress you are subject to.

Treatment begins as an overall massage to relax the foot and the patient. Any deposits which are located at this stage are noted for further intensive attention. Concentration on areas which have accumulated a deposit will take place over a course of treatment, usually six sessions. During this time you may notice your skin worsens as the body eliminates toxins. Such after-effects show that the therapy is working, and do not last long.

Reflexology And Arthritis

If you are planning to administer reflexology to yourself, or to someone else, you will need to attend a seminar to learn the position of the zones and the correct techniques to use. There is, for example, a particular head and sinuses technique which involves 'walking' the thumb of one hand down each of the toes on the opposite foot, and similarly, there are specific areas to alleviate the pain of arthritis and rheumatism. These may include stimulating, or dampening, the actions of the pituitary gland, the solar plexus and the adrenal glands. Additionally, depending on where your arthritis is sited, those particular areas will need to be identified on the feet.

There are documented cases where patients have had their operations for a joint replacement cancelled as a result of a course of reflexology to relieve the pain! However, such incidences are rare and you should only consider reflexology as a natural, safe way to ease your pain while you take other steps to treat your arthritis.

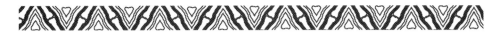

Finding A Practitioner

For more information, write, enclosing a SAE, to the Council for Acupuncture, 38 Mount Pleasant, London WC1X OAP.

The British Reflexology Association, 12 Pond Road, London SE3 9JL, maintains a register of members which is updated three times a year. Its official teaching body is the Bayley School of Reflexology.

Further Reading

Acupressure: Headway Lifeguides by Eliana Harvey and Mary Jane Oatley (Headway)

Acupressure's Potent Points by Michael Reed Gach (Bantam Books)

Reflexology: A Definitive Guide to Self-Treatment by Chris Stormer (Headway)

Reflexology: Headway Lifeguides by Chris Stormer (Headway)

The Art of Reflexology by Inge Dougans with Suzanne Ellis (Element)

The Reflexology and Colour Therapy Workbook by Pauline Wills (Element)

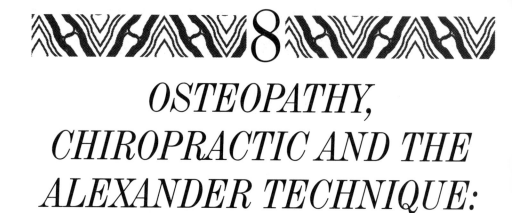

OSTEOPATHY, CHIROPRACTIC AND THE ALEXANDER TECHNIQUE: BODY WORK

The fundamental tenet of osteopathy, according to its founder, Andrew Still, is that the body has an inbuilt mechanism to heal itself. He therefore developed a method to deal with the structural malfunctions and misalignments that prevent the body from performing its proper function of healing and repair. Health problems which relate to the degeneration of one or more of our body systems can benefit a great deal from osteopathic treatment since it will assist in the body's own repair mechanism. Further, osteopathic treatment can also help by ensuring that the peripheral strains on the body interfere as little as possible with the healing process. In the case of arthritis, while osteopathy cannot repair the worn cartilage surface, gentle stretching exercises can do much to relieve pain and help regain joint flexibility to a great degree.

The Origins And Theory Of Osteopathy

Andrew Taylor Still was born in 1828 in Virginia, USA. He became disenchanted with the then current medical practices after the deaths of his three children. Trained as an engineer, later as a physician, he practised medicine in the army. Applying the trained logic of an engineer, he reasoned that illness should be treated for its causes and not simply its symptoms. Still's studies of the interdependence of the body's structure (loss of movement may be the cause of back pain, a trapped nerve in the neck may be the cause of pain in the wrist or shoulder, for example) and his Christian beliefs (he was a minister's son) led him to conclude that the human body contained the ability to heal itself, and that the body must be viewed in its entirety as a complete unit. Still's

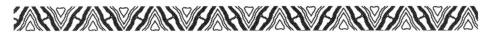

approach to medicine, then, was holisitic. His theory of osteopathy (he coined the name himself) is based on three principles:

- the normal, healthy body has its own innate powers of healing and defence mechanisms;
- the body is a unit and one malfunctioning part of it will have effects on other parts of the body;
- the body is in its optimum state of operation when it has maximum structural mobility and flexibility.

On this last principle, Still has sometimes been misquoted and misunderstood. He did not mean that all disease stems from problems of the spine or of the skeleton as a whole. What he did mean was that the skeleton, as the body's structure, has a cause and effect on the health of the rest of the body, its muscles, blood system and joints.

Osteopathy as a medical practice became widely accepted and practised in the US and today its validity is recognised worldwide.

A Modern Osteopath

Osteopathy in Still's time was used to cure any and all of the body's ills. Today osteopathy largely confines itself to the treatment of problems of the spine, ligaments, muscles, bones; it also promotes lymphatic drainage and improves breathing.

A visit to an osteopath begins with taking a detailed case-history, followed by an examination of the whole spine, including the problem area. The patient's posture and ease of mobility will be studied from the moment of entering the consulting room. The muscles, joints and entire surface of the body are examined to reveal any problem areas which may need gentle correction. The osteopath does not seek to transform every patient's skeleton into a blueprint of perfection – this would be medically impossible, in any case. An osteopath's aim is to enable the body to work as efficiently as possible for the individual concerned.

Joint manipulation

The most popularly known use of osteopathy is the manipulation of joints. What is commonly called 'joint cracking' is termed 'high velocity thrust' (HVT) by osteopaths. Contrary to popular belief, the crack of the manipulation has nothing to do with a dislocated

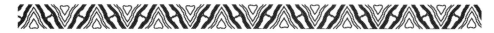

bone being put back into position. As we have seen earlier, the synovial joints are enclosed in a fibrous capsule which is lined with the synovial membrane. The joint surfaces are held together by partial vacuum. Therefore the pressure inside the capsule is slightly lower than the outside atmospheric pressure. When the joint is manipulated the joint surfaces are separated slightly. As this disturbs the normal pressure inside the capsule, tiny bubbles of gas are released which cause the popping sound. However, it it is not the popping sound, nor the release of the bubbles, that relieves pain. In fact the osteopath's aim is to stretch the joint capsule in order to relieve pain and improve the mobility of the joint.

Treatment

There is no standard treatment as most osteopaths believe individual treatment has to be created for each patient according to the patient's condition. There are various self-help techniques, such as Muscle Energy Technique (MET), which can help deal with day-to-day sprains and strains. An excellent book by Leon Chaitow '*Osteopathic Self-Treatment' (Thorsons)* has detailed techniques which augment rather than replace professional treatment. Needless-to-say, care should be taken before embarking upon such a course and self-treatment should only be used when the cause of the problem has been identified.

Chiropractic

Of all the manipulative therapies, chiropractic is probably the most similar to osteopathy. Chiropractic, like osteopathy, is a manipulative therapy, and their techniques are therefore similar. However, osteopathy concentrates on the movement of the joints and uses leverage more than chiropractic, whilst chiropractic places greater emphasis on direct contact on the spine's vertebrae for their adjustment. Chiropractic works more on the spine and its effects on the nervous system and related effects on the rest of the body; X-rays are used in diagnosis.

Chiropractic treats backache, neck pain and low backache, by gentle manipulation of the spine. The theory is that, since the spine has nerves radiating off it which reach every part of the body, the spine is the key to eliminating pain in the whole body. A displaced vertebra, for example, puts pressure on a nerve which may result in

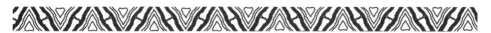

pain in a limb or give rise to a headache. The chiropractor uses his skill to discover which vertebra is misaligned and then corrects it. No drugs are used, since chiropractic is entirely manipulative. Chiropractors specialise in diagnosing and treating problems of the spine, joints or muscles.

An initial consultation with a chiropractor will feature an in-depth historical analysis to include childhood injuries and current lifestyle. A thorough physical examination is conducted, including a routine examination such as you would receive from a GP. A manipulative examination of the muscles, skin, bone and joints reveals to the chiropractor whether chiropractic is in fact suitable for your problem or if you should be referred back to your GP. That said, the manipulative examination explores the texture, tenderness and movement of the body from which the chiropractor makes his diagnosis. X-rays form part of the examination. Thinning of the bones, infective arthritis and other malformations such as bony growths in the joints are all clearly shown on X-ray films.

If chiropractic is called for, treatment techniques might include massage of the muscles and ligaments, stretching of ligaments, instruction on posture, rotary massage and direct localised pressure on the troubled body part. Depending on the scale of the medical problem, benefits may be apparent after only one session, or several appointments may be necessary.

The basic chiropractic manipulation, usually known as *adjustment*, is similar to cracking the knuckles. When a sharp thrust is applied to the joints, the sudden separation of surfaces (lined by flexible tissue which has a thin film of fluid) produces a sound that is akin to the sound produced when a wet rubber sucker is pulled off a glass surface.

Treatment

Chiropractors find that cases of arthritis can be helped by restoring function to the joints and believe that the real cause of the condition is stiffness of the vertebral joints themselves. In June 1990 the British Medical Journal published results of a three-year trial by the Medical Research Council which compared chiropractic treatment for back pain with hospital out-patient treatment. It was found that chiropractic was 70 per cent more effective.

Chiropractic manipulations are not suitable for self-treatment since manipulation is a precise technique and should be done by a professional.

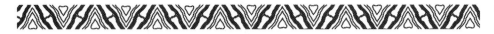

The Alexander Technique

Teachers of the Alexander Technique believe you can learn to improve your posture so that your body is able to work in a more natural, released and efficient manner. The technique is entirely safe, promotes a harmonious state of both mind and body, and helps a number of medical conditions, including arthritis and rheumatism.

The method was developed by an Australian actor, Frederick Matthias Alexander, who found himself losing his voice on stage and discovered that he could cure the problem by improving his posture. He realised that the relationship between the head, neck and back was vitally important for good health. His discovery became the basis for a whole technique for retraining the body's movements and positions. Today there are Alexander training schools and teachers all over the world.

Learning the technique

'Lessons' are usually given on a one-to-one basis. The 'teacher' begins by watching how you use your body. Even simple activities such as walking or reading a book involve the use of many muscles, and a certain amount of muscular tension and 'spring' is needed just to react against the pull of gravity. Children move naturally, but so often acquire bad habits as they grow up. Stress is created in such simple actions as holding a pen too tightly or clenching the jaw while opening a jam jar. Excess stress on the joints seems to play a part in causing arthritis. The hips, spine, knees and hands are the parts most affected. They lose the mobility of their design.

Glynn Macdonald, a highly experienced teacher of the Alexander Technique and author of *The Alexander Technique* (Headway), writes,

> 'In order to get the benefit of being light and springy, we have to stop tightening and collapsing, by allowing the head and all the joints of the body to work more freely. Every bone in the body forms a joint with some other bone. Without joints we could make no movements at all, our bodies would be rigid and immobile. The joints are designed to release and expand, but often we hinder this ability by becoming rigid and inflexible, and pain can result.'

Some people suffer from chronic muscular tension, which throws the head, neck and back out of alignment, causing rounded shoulders, a bowed head, stiff joints and arched back. If this is not corrected, the spine develops a curve and a hump may appear at the

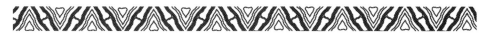

base of the neck. This causes back pain and puts a strain on the heart, lungs and digestive system and on the joints. Breathing can be restricted and poor circulation can develop. If you correct these problems of posture, the joints have a chance to become less painful.

The Alexander teacher shows you how to stop these harmful habits and how to begin to use muscles with minimum effort and maximum efficiency. While you stand, sit or lie down, the teacher gently manipulates your body into a more efficient and effective way of being, while explaining to you where you are going wrong. Gradually, by constant practising and thinking about how you perform even the simplest actions, you should learn to release tension and use your body correctly. The teacher uses no force and there is no wrenching or clicking of joints – just a subtle adjustment as you learn to walk, sit, stand and move all over again, in a free, released way.

Lessons last about 30 or 45 minutes, and a course of 30 is usual, after which you should have learnt the basics.

Finding A Practitioner

For a list of practitioners or further information write, sending a SAE to:

Osteopathy
The General Council and Register of Osteopaths, 56 London Street, Reading, Berkshire RG14BQ;

The British Naturopathy and Osteopathy Association, 6 Netherall Gardens, London NW3 5RR;

Chiropractic
The British Chiropractic Association, 29 Whitley Street, Reading, Berkshire RG2 2EG; Telephone Freephone 0800 212618 for your nearest practitioner.

The Institute of Pure Chiropractic, 14 Park End Street, Oxford OX2 1HH;

Alexander Technique
Society of Teachers of the Alexander Technique (STAT), 10 Station House, 266 Fulham Road, London SW10 9EL.

Further Reading

Alexander Technique: Headway Lifeguides by Glynn Macdonald
   (Headway)
Chiropractic by S Moore (Macdonald Optima)
Chiropractic Today by Copland-Griffiths (Thorsons)
Osteopathy Self Treatment by Leon Chaitow (Thorsons)

9

AROMATHERAPY: SCENT FOR JOINT HEALTH

The word 'aromatherapy' is itself a clue as to the aim of the technique. 'Aromatherapy' combines the words 'aroma', thus recognising the importance of smell, and 'therapy'. Essential oils from plants are used to stimulate the sensory organs, and a particular type of massage is sometimes given at the same time.

Aromatherapy is not a new therapy. The earliest surviving text describing the use of plant essences for healing is Chinese and is dated 1000–700 BC. The Bible also describes the healing power of plants and their essences. The ancient Egyptians, too, used aromatic oils for medicinal purposes and embalming and when the tomb of Tutankhamun was opened the faint smell of aromatic oils was still detectable. The Romans used plant essences for cookery and medicine and they are credited with introducing aromatherapy to Britain.

During the Middle Ages the study of medicine declined in Europe but in Asia it flourished. Abu Ibn Sina (AD 982), or Avicenna, to give him his Western name, was an Arab physician and philosopher who developed a technique of steam distillation for extracting essences from plants and made aromatherapy a viable treatment. This extraction method is still used today.

During the European Renaissance (the great revival of art, literature and learning in Europe in the fourteenth, fifteenth and sixteenth centuries) new plant species were introduced to Europe and the following centuries saw an increase in the extraction and use of essential oils for antiseptics, perfumes and medicines.

The Industrial Revolution during the nineteenth century heralded the age of chemistry and chemical substitutes brought a decline in the use of plants and their essences until it was found that these substitutes were not effective in the same way as their natural models. (Each essential oil is a complex mixture of organic substances, and its therapeutic value depends on not just one of its constituents, but on the whole delicate mixture. The number of constituents in essential oil make it impossible to make exact chemical copies.)

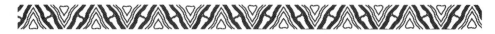

It was not until a French doctor, René Gattefosse (1881-1950), accidentally discovered the healing power of lavender oil that aromatherapy was reborn. Working in his laboratory one day, he burned his hand and plunged it into the nearest available liquid, which happened to be essential lavender oil. When his hand healed extremely rapidly and without trace of a scar, he was intrigued by the therapeutic effects of lavender oil. His subsequent research led to the widespread use of aromatherapy, even to the extent of its usage to heal wounded soldiers during the First World War. The name *aromatherapy* was coined by Gattefosse.

After Gattefosse's death, his work was continued by the French physician Jean Valnet who used essential oils of clove, lemon and chamomile as natural disinfectants and antiseptics to fumigate hospital wards and to sterilise surgical instruments. The link between aromatherapy and the cosmetic industry was forged and developed by a French biochemist, Marguerite Maury (1895-1968), who was instrumental in developing the aromatherapeutic massage techniques.

What Are Essential Oils?

Essential oils are found in all plants and herbs to produce fragrance or flavour. The oils are extracted from all the parts of a plant – the flowers, leaves, stems, roots and rinds of fruit.

Extraction Techniques

The most common method is steam distillation as invented by Abu Ibn Sina: pressurised steam is passed through the plant, the heat evaporates the oil which is then condensed by passing through a water cooler. Solvents are another method of extraction: a solvent, such as petrol ether, is sprayed on the plant and evaporated off to leave behind the oil. The oils of fruit are extracted by expression: the rinds are pressed or grated and the oils from the torn cells are collected in a sponge and squeezed out.

The quantity of plants required to produce essential oils is staggering: 70 kg of plants yield, on average, just 1 kg of essential oil. The season and even the time of the day that the plant is harvested affect the final yield quantity. For example, jasmine harvested at sunset will yield the greatest amount of oil, as it is a night-scented flower. The rose, meanwhile, has so little oil that it may take 100 kg

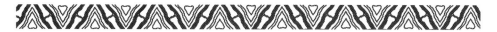

of some varieties of rose petals to make up to half a litre of oil. The final price of the essential oil depends on yield, which is why rose is the most expensive of the essential oils.

How Essential Oils Work

The oils are chemically complex, with hundreds of substances chemically active – some of the substances are understood but many more are not. What has come to light as a result of the attempted chemical synthesisation of the oils is that it is not possible to extract just one of the hundreds of chemically active substances and feel the benefits. For example, the known active substance in lemongrass is aldehyde citral; when chemically synthesised it produces an allergic reaction when applied to the skin. However, natural lemongrass oil does not produce any such allergic reaction and testing has shown that the other constituents in natural lemongrass oil neutralise the harmful effects of aldehyde citral.

All the oils are antiseptics and stimulate the immune system. As well as their specific therapeutic qualities, the essential oils are believed to promote a sense of physical and mental well-being.

In all cases, the oils are effective by entering the bloodstream. This can happen in a variety of ways. When massaged into the skin, the oils diffuse into the capillaries (delicate blood vessels) and thence enter the main bloodstream. The massage itself stimulates the blood circulation, and the immune system, thus building up the body's resistance to disease. Massage also soothes tense, painful muscles and induces a relaxed physical and mental state. Some aromatherapists use the same pressure points that are used in acupuncture or acupressure: in this way particular organs as well as the entire body receive the benefit. On an emotional level, touch is one of our five senses, and it is a powerful and effective means of communication. Young babies and children need the reassurance of a hug from their parents to feel that they are loved and cared for; a fact which still carries over, albeit to a lesser extent, in adult life, but which we tend to neglect. Massage instils a sense of being cared for and loved, and in this way it attends to our emotional needs.

The oils have either a tonic or a sedative effect when used in baths: the pores open and the oils enter the bloodstream that way, and they are also inhaled and thus pass into the lungs and from there into the bloodstream. Baths relax the muscles and therefore promote relaxation and stress relief.

When a few drops of essential oils are placed on a handkerchief and inhaled, or placed in a room diffuser, the oils pass directly into the bloodstream via the lungs. A diffuser is a small earthenware or china container designed to burn off essential oils over several hours. On top there is a shallow receptacle into which a little water and a few drops of the essential oils are placed. Directly underneath there is a small candle. The heat from the candle warms the oil and its aroma is released into the room. Diffusers are increasingly available, together with essential oils, from high street stores and chemists.

Different smells affect us in different ways. They can trigger memories and act on the subconscious. The olfactory nerves, those which affect our sense of smell, affect memory, thinking and behaviour. We all know that we respond with pleasure to some smells, and with disgust to others. This may explain how aromatherapy helps with the emotional or mental aspects of healing. Different smells may be used to relax or stimulate, depending on the needs of the patient.

Aromatherapy And Stress Relief

Stress-related illnesses are an ever-increasing health problem, from everyday ailments, such as headaches, to the more serious ailments, such as arthritis and rheumatism. Stress impairs the action of the immune system and the body's resistance to illness is therefore compromised. However, stress itself is not the problem but a person's inability to cope with it. Dealing with stress in its early stages can prevent serious illnesses. Aromatherapy can be regarded as a preventative therapy since it emphasises the importance of dealing with stress.

The combination of massage and essential oils is particularly effective. The essential oils work on mental tension while massage alleviates physical tension. The effects of an aromatic massage often include dramatic improvements in sleeping patterns, leading to heightened vitality and physical energy. Consequently, stress-related disorders, such as digestive problems, acne and skin disorders and tensed muscles and joints, can be treated effectively with aromatherapy. This is partly due to the release of mood-inducing chemicals in the brain and body which act as either stimulants or sedatives. Some essential oils trigger the release of natural painkillers, with obvious benefits.

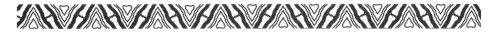

Essential Oils For Arthritis And Rheumatism

Since RA is the effect of the body's overactive immune function, drugs are usually given to dampen the immune system's activity. There are no essential oils which have this effect; on the contrary, specific oils will increase the immune system's activity and these must therefore be avoided. However, the use of massage with muscle relaxing oils will be beneficial.

OA, as we have seen can be caused either by mechanical stress on the joints and bones, or by an infection. If the joints continue to be stressed, inflammation around the joint and cartilage disintegration will occur until the joint is so damaged that a replacement joint may be the only option. To prevent such a serious development, massage of the joints and stimulation of the blood circulation are beneficial. At the same time, care must be taken not to overwork the affected joint and a nutritious diet should be adopted (see Chapter 3). If the cause is due to an infection, oils to boost the immune system will be required.

- *Lavender* boosts the immune system and has an antiseptic effect, and is therefore suitable. It also boosts the circulatory system, so encouraging the supply of oxygen-rich blood to muscles and ensuring that nutrients are distributed through the body. On the emotional and mental levels, lavender has a sedative, calming effect. Depending on the severity of pain, massage may or may not be possible on the areas which are affected, but in this case an overall massage will still give the benefits of promoting relaxation and improved circulation.
- At one time *chamomile* was used in hospitals for its powerful antiseptic effects; it is especially beneficial for OA since it stimulates the immune system. Consequently, it should *not* be used in RA. Where arthritis is the result of infection, chamomile is very beneficial since it will encourage the destruction of harmful bacteria. Used in a bath, compress or massage, chamomile will ease inflammations of the joints or muscles.
- *Cypress* can be used safely for all types of arthritis since it does not specifically stimulate the immune system. It does improve blood circulation and, as an astringent, can reduce excess acids which, if they are a contributory factor to your type of arthritis, will doubly benefit you. Cypress eases nervous tension and relaxes the body and mind.
- *Pine* combined with cypress has a powerful antiseptic effect. On its own, it treats infections and improves blood circulation. Used in a hot compress it will relieve the affected area, or alternatively a few drops in a warm bath will treat the entire body.

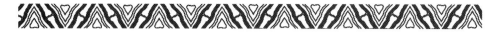

- *Juniper* is safe for all types of arthritis. It should be used to massage the stiff joints, or in a compress, or in a warm bath. Juniper is a diuretic which, if fluid retention has caused a weight increase, will be beneficial. Attention to weight is important in OA to avoid strain on the affected joints. Juniper is a powerful cleanser, tonic and antiseptic agent, all of which will help to reduce and eliminate an infection.
- *Eucalyptus* has been well known for centuries for its antiseptic properties. However, it also stimulates the immune system, and therefore should *not* be used for RA. For OA eucalyptus combines its qualities of antiseptic and stimulant to reduce infection and improve a sluggish blood circulation and/or immune system. Use it in a compress applied directly to the affected joint, or in a bath, or in a massage.
- *Coriander*, more familiar to us from Indian cuisine, is easily faked by a mixture of other oils, and so care must be taken to buy it from a reputable source. *Note that an overdose can be toxic, even fatal. So, use very sparingly.* However, coriander is very effective in reducing inflammations, in stimulating the blood supply and in pain relief. Consult a qualified aromatherapist for guidance on dosage and usage.
- *Lemon*, with its crisp, clean aroma, stimulates the immune system and should *not* be used for RA. Lemon detoxifies and purifies the blood and its antiseptic qualities destroy harmful bacteria. It is also a diuretic and so may help weight loss.
- The qualities of essential *rosemary* oil will vary. The cheaper oils are taken from the stems and leaves, before the plant flowers, but the best and more expensive essential rosemary oil is taken from the flowers themselves. Rosemary oil is a strong antiseptic and stimulates the circulation of blood. It relaxes stiff muscles and joints and relieves aches and pains generally. Use it in a bath, compress or massage to benefit from its effects. Rosemary blends well with lavender to combine their qualities. However, because it stimulates the lymph system, it must *not* be used in cases of RA.
- *Marjoram* combined with rosemary is effective in relieving muscle inflammation and pain from strained muscles and bruised joints. It is also a gentle sedative, relieving nervous tension and stress and is comforting and warming. Use it in a bath, massage, compress or diffuser.
- *Ginger* has a warming effect, much like a heat rub. Its application to painful muscles will soon bring relief. Use it in a bath or compress to stimulate the blood circulation and relieve all types of arthritic pain. Care should be taken in not overdosing, as this herb can increase the surface temperature of the skin to uncomfortable levels.

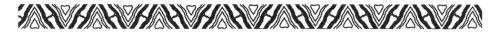

Summary

Aromatherapy, then, can relieve arthritis in various ways. It can relieve stress and tension, which cause further damage to the joints. It can help to increase the blood circulation and thus prevent the joints from seizing up. It can stimulate the immune system and improve the body's ability to fight off the infection which may have caused the arthritis. It can reduce the painful inflammations and swellings. Above all, perhaps, aromatherapy can soothe irritated emotions and make the process of healing an enjoyable experience which can be carried out in your own home.

Of course, it would be foolish to claim that aromatherapy itself can cure arthritis and your doctor will need to monitor your progress with conventional treatment. But aromatherapy can bring much physical and emotional relief from the debilitating effects of arthritis and, if you have not contracted the disease, help to ensure that you do not fall prey to it at all.

In Conversation With An Aromatherapist

Q. Can aromatherapy be used to treat all types of illnesses and conditions, or are there limitations?
A.This is a difficult question to answer, as it varies not only from practitioner to practitioner, but from country to country. In France, for example, doctors use aromatherapy for a variety of ailments, and even prescribe essential oils for internal use – in the same way as conventional doctors use drugs.

In this country, though, the majority of aromatherapists are not medically trained, so they tend to just concentrate on aromatherapy as a means of reducing stress – which in itself can trigger a healing effect. This is just my approach, though: other aromatherapists would say, 'Yes, aromatherapy can treat any condition'. In theory, aromatherapy can be used to treat any illness.

Q. Can anyone treat themselves using aromatherapy, at home, even for quite serious illnesses?
A. I wouldn't say serious illnesses. No, you would need help from a holistic practitioner who would take an overall look at your illness and your whole lifestyle – otherwise you are just treating the illness symptomatically which would never really do much. For instance, if you have athlete's foot

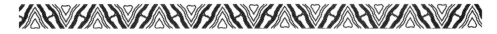

you can put lavender oil on it and it may go away, but on the other hand it may come back again — in which case you're never actually doing anything to address the cause which may be not just the effect of feet enclosed in trainers, perhaps, but a symptom of stress, vitamin B deficiency, whatever. There may be a need for deeper treatment — a look at your diet, taking garlic capsules, and so on. You can treat minor ailments at home but if it doesn't work, and they keep coming back, it may be necessary to look deeper.

Q. Can aromatherapy be used safely in conjunction with other therapies, such as acupuncture, homoeopathy and conventional drug treatment?
A. With acupuncture, I don't think there is a problem, although again this depends on the practitioner. Some acupuncturists would say that it's best if you just have one treatment at a time, otherwise you don't know which treatment is working. Otherwise, I think that gentle massage with a very low dilution of oil wouldn't do any harm at all — and I think it would be harmonious, because it's all about balance.

   With homoeopathy, again, some homoeopaths are very strict about using any aromatics — even toothpaste will act as an antidote to some of the remedies, whereas some homoeopaths disagree, so there really isn't any definitive answer. But, traditionally, eucalyptus and peppermint, and perhaps camphor, have been known to antidote some homoeopathic medicines, as does coffee, simply because it is so aromatic. It's best to ask the homoeopath.

Q. As a practising aromatherapist, would you be happy for a patient to undergo homoeopathic treatment or acupuncture at the same time as taking essential oils?
A. Yes, as long as not too many treatments are mixed at the same time. Massage in general is such a good relaxant it enhances the internal conditions which help to trigger our immune defences.

Q. Talking about massage, it wasn't until this century that massage was introduced as a part of aromatherapy treatment — how crucial is it to aromatherapy?
A. Before Marguerite Maury's use of massage in the 1950s, doctors tended to use essential oils as simply another form of herbal medicine to treat external conditions. Mood-enhancing herbs were used by the ancient Egyptians but not as essential oils because techniques of distillation were not yet discovered.

   In France, doctors do not use massage very much — Marguerite Maury

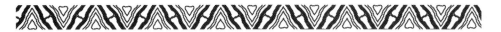

brought the technique to this country. Massage is about the most important part of the therapy in this country as a means of relieving stress, and this is the area which most interests me. Most illness is the result of disharmony of the emotions and the mind.

Q. Are there any scientific studies into the effects of aromatherapy and its healing powers?
A. Yes. In France and Germany it has been very widely researched. Recently German scientists have found that frankincense contains the same substances as cannabis, so there is evidence to show that there is a mood-enhancing substance in it.

Q. In this country essential oils are commonly available: are there any guidelines to purchasing oils?
A. It's best to get to know the oils with a practised nose, so that you buy the pure essential oils; very often they are too diluted for traditional dosages to be of benefit. Buy from well-established herbal houses from health food shops. The International Federation of Aromatherapists may advise on where to purchase.

Q. How do the essential oils boost the immune system?
A. They release endorphins, for example, which make us feel happy – but all pleasures in life have this effect. Of course, when we are happy we are less likely to become ill. Thyme, chamomile and lavender are widely used in France to boost white cell production. Aromatherapy is a multifaceted therapy which works on many levels. It boosts our own healing mechanisms on a physical and emotional level.

Q. Are there any conditions which must not use essential oils, for example, asthma or serious heart conditions?
A. Some essential oils can be hazardous in pregnancy or in particular conditions or allergies. Please consult a qualified aromatherapist before proceeding with any self-treatment.

Q. What is meant by 'strong' oils?
A. Ginger is a strong oil, a 'rubefacient' – it causes redness in the skin which is part of its healing properties (the idea is to bring warmth into the area but to some people that redness may flare up into a rash if you use it in a very high concentration). All oils are diluted, never used neat. Dilutions vary according to the strength of the oil – ginger would be only one drop in 20 ml of oil, whereas if you use lavender you can use three drops per teaspoon. No two oils are the same.

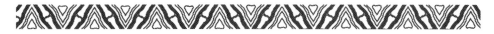

Q. How much experience is necessary to use essential oils?
A. If you have no experience, keep to very low concentrations and avoid the known potentially risky oils — clove oil is one which should never be used directly on the skin, for example.

Q. How long does it take to train as an aromatherapist?
A. There are a number of courses; qualifications in anatomy and physiology are necessary and a good course will last at least a year. But at the moment the law in this country does not demand any qualifications before a person sets up as a practising aromatherapist — some people just attend a weekend course and set up in practice, although they would not be on the list of the International Register of Aromatherapists.

Q. Where do you place aromatherapy in the field of healing?
A. In my opinion, aromatherapists should only see themselves in a complementary field, that is, to aid the person's own healing mechanisms, and to promote relaxation. Holistic therapy is not about treating a condition but the whole person.

Q. What would you say is the most important healing aspect of aromatherapy?
A. The tender loving care which an aromatherapist provides!

Finding An Aromatherapist

For a list of practitioners or further information write, sending a SAE to:

International Federation of Aromatherapists, Department of Continuing Education, Royal Masonic Hospital, Ravenscourt Park, London W6 OTN;

Aromatherapy Organisations Council, 3 Latymer Close, Braybrooke, Market Harborough, Leicestershire LE16 8LN.

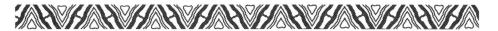

Further Reading

Aromatherapy: Headway Lifeguides by Denise Brown (Headway)
Aromatherapy by Daniele Ryman (Piatkus)
Aromatherapy: A Definitive Guide To Essential Oils by Lisa Chidell
(Headway)
Aromatherapy – Massage With Essential Oils by Christine Wildwood
(Element Books)
The Art of Aromatherapy by Robert Tisserand (C W Daniel)

10

CONCLUSION

Does it make a difference which of the therapies, orthodox or complementary, you choose to attain health and well-being? There is no simple answer to this. If you are looking to eliminate the symptoms of your disorder as opposed to healing mind, body and spirit, then any therapy that quickly and effectively deals with the symptom would be acceptable. However, if you consider healing as attaining health and being wholly well again, then you have to look at all the therapies in a very different light.

Healing does not mean that since the body has malfunctioned then we go and repair it. When the body malfunctions, it has an effect on us at various levels. If I say I have a headache, it means that the pain in me as a person is manifesting itself in my head. If I just treat the head by, for example, taking aspirin, it means I am disregarding the source of inner pain.

Neither the GP and her drugs, nor the herbalist and his herbs, nor the aromatherapist and her essential oils, nor the acupuncturist and his needles, nor the osteopath and her manipulation, and not even the anthroposophical doctor with his art therapy, eurythmy and hydrotherapy can heal. Only you can heal yourself. 'Each patient carries his own doctor inside him,' said Dr Albert Schweitzer.

In order to begin the process of healing you must want to achieve health. This means the will to get better is of supreme importance and consequently it has to be acknowledged that the mind–body interaction comes into play.

A cognisance of this body–mind interaction will result in an integration of the body and the mind in the process of achieving wellness. That is what healing is all about. If this is understood, then it is easy to understand why the therapies described in this book can be effective. Whatever therapy we may choose, it can only be effective if we have a positive attitude towards the healing technique and the person who helps us to heal ourselves.

The culture of dependency spawned by modern medical intervention, of curing the sick parts of the body, has conditioned us to lose faith in our ability to heal ourselves. We have come to rely on medication as a form of reassurance and believe that the prescription will 'cure'.

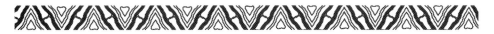

The root of this thinking could be attributed to René Descartes whose dictum, 'I think therefore I am', crystallised the concept of separating *res cognitas* (the realm of the mind) and *res extensa* (the realm of matter). His perception of the material world has so permeated our culture that we now view the human body as an elaborate machine made up of assembled parts.

Descartes said, 'I consider the human body as a machine. My thought compares the sick man and an ill-made clock with my idea of a healthy man and a well-made clock.' This legacy of dualism has guided and moulded the basis of modern medicine up to the present time.

Indeed, the study of disease has focused on biological processes, attributing the causes of all illness to biological factors. Modern medicine, preoccupied with measurements, statistical models and double-blind crossover studies, fails to take into account the person as a whole and sometimes appears to preclude the human potential for self-healing. The mind–body relationship has sometimes been ignored in healing. Whatever the disease, unless we accept that this relationship does exist it is not possible to achieve true healing or true health and well-being.

We must first recognise that mind and body are both aspects of the human whole; that they are interrelated and cannot be seen in isolation from each other. The state of perfect balance between mind and body, as sometimes experienced in childhood, can be achieved.

To do that, we have to understand the role of the mind and the body working and affecting each other. There is a complex system of information that conveys messages between the mind and the body contained in our bloodstream.

Regulation by the *pituitary gland* (a gland, attached to the brain, which releases hormones) and the *hypothalamus* (a region of the brain situated between the eyes which has nerve connections from all over the nervous system) controls the psychological and emotional activity in relation to the physical function of the body. A good example of such a connection is the *vegas nerve* which links the stomach to the hypothalamus; hence stress or anxiety can cause stomach upsets.

We have seen that the immune system is indispensable for defence against disease-causing substances. However, we can be left vulnerable to disease if certain hormones are released by the adrenal glands which disrupt the relationship between the brain and

the immune system. In addition to stress, this disruption can be caused by repressed feelings such as prolonged anger, bitterness and other negative emotions and thoughts.

The *limbic system* (a ring shaped area in the brain) consists of clusters of nerve cells, including the hypothalamus. Called the 'seat of emotions', the limbic system regulates the *autonomic nervous functions*, such as sweating, digestion and heart rate, and has a bearing on our emotions and sense of smell. The limbic system is therefore important in the body–mind relationship. This, in turn, is influenced by the *cerebral cortex* (the part of the brain responsible for thinking, perception, memory and all other intellectual activity).

Stress is an example of the result of the alarm sounded by the cerebral cortex when it perceives a life-threatening situation. As soon as the alarm bells ring, the limbic system, and consequently the nervous system and the immune system, are all galvanised into action. The reaction is tense muscles, constricted blood vessels and other symptoms that set into motion a general nervous disarray.

Some reactions are instantaneous, such as blushing when the emotions produce the effect of blood rushing to the face; others, such as repressed anger, are cumulative and take longer to manifest themselves in the form of disease.

There is little doubt that there is an innate link between the mind and the body, each affecting the other. Negative thoughts and emotions will result in weakened defences which will lead to disease and, ultimately, death. Our recognition of the body–mind connection is reflected in our everyday language when we say, 'He is eaten up with jealousy', or 'His heart is broken', or 'The stress is killing him', or 'He is worn down with grief', or 'She is radiantly happy'.

Most of the traditional healing disciplines, based on different world views and cosmological principles, have a common thread: they deal with illness by considering humans in the context of their relationship with the cosmos.

Traditionally, Muslim doctors have regarded their patients as integrated entities of mind, body and spirit with a vital force.

The Yogic view of the human body is that it is composed of three different manifestations: the physical body (composed of flesh, blood and bone), the subtle body (containing the life force *prana*) and the spiritual body (which encompasses universal wisdom).

To the Hawaiians, health means energy. Good health is a state of *ehuehu* (abundant energy) and poor health is *pake* (weakness).

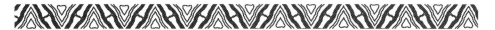

Illness is caused by *mai* (tension) and healing is equated to the restoration of *lapau* (energy). Health therefore is 'a state of harmonious energy'.

The American Indians consider that *Earth Mother* is a living organism, and that all creations on this earth contain a life force and are part of a harmonious whole. Illness occurs when this balance is upset and the purpose of healing ceremonies is to restore both personal and universal harmony.

Tai Chi is the Chinese way of increasing the energy flow in the body and strengthening the body's resistance to disease. Tai Chi is thought to stimulate the kidney (seen as the life force energy) and to maintain vitality of mind, body and spirit.

Rudolf Steiner, the founder of anthroposophy (see Chapter 6), sought to go beyond the idea of healing the body. His acute perception led him to explore the spiritual side of existence which resulted in an understanding of the ways of stimulating the natural healing forces in the person. Healing was a matter of considering the interrelation between the four aspects of the human being (the physical body, the etheric body, the astral body and the ego) and treating them as a whole.

There are striking similarities in the various healing systems reviewed above. Call it by any name – *prana, rooh, chi*, life force, *ehuehu*, etheric energy – we all have it in us. It is up to the 'doctor inside', to borrow Albert Schweitzer's phrase, to harness this healing force within us and so to achieve that state of balance between body, mind and spirit.

Of late the holistic approach to health care has begun to gain momentum. The proponents of this model have gone some way to counter the mechanistic and reductionist streaks in modern medicine. Holism is based on the premise that the human organism is a multidimensional being, possessing body, mind and spirit, all inextricably linked and that disease results from an imbalance either from within or from an external force. The human body possesses a powerful and innate capacity to heal itself by bringing itself back into a state of balance. The primary task of the practitioner is to encourage and assist the body in its attempts to heal itself. The practitioner's role is that of an educator rather than an interventionist.

The true test of healing must surely be a practical manifestation of harmony between the mind, the body and the spirit. Holism has some answers but matters of the spirit, while acknowledged, are

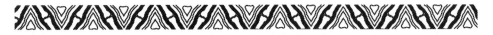

avoided in practice. Yet without the spiritual dimension no system of healing can be truly whole. Holism may acknowledge the spirit 'in spirit' but this dimension remains untouched. Without it, however, no system can be whole. There can be no true self-healing and no true holistic medicine.

You picked up this book because you or a loved one suffers from rheumatism or arthritis and because you have an open mind, you are willing to explore different types of interaction between the body and the mind. **You** are responsible for drawing spirit into the equation and the final message of this book is that so-called 'holism' that looks only at the mind and the body, ignoring the spirit, is an illusion – go for a truer reality and use this book as, perhaps, a first step on the road to uniting body, mind and spirit.

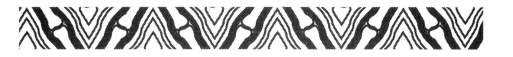

GLOSSARY

Acute Symptom that comes on suddenly, usually for a short period.

Adrenaline Hormone released by the adrenal gland, triggered by fear or stress.

Allergy A condition caused by the reaction of the immune system to a specific substance.

Allopathy A term used to describe conventional drug-based medicine.

Amino acids A group of chemical compounds containing nitrogen that form the basic building blocks in the production of protein. Of the 22 known amino acids, 8 are considered essential because they cannot be made by the body and therefore must be obtained from the diet.

Anaemia A condition that results when there is a low level of red blood cells.

Analgesic A substance that relieves pain.

Antibiotic A medication that helps to treat infection caused by bacteria.

Antibody Protein molecule released by the body's immune system that neutralises or counteracts foreign organisms.

Antidote A substance that neutralises or counteracts the effects of a poison.

Antigen Any substance that can trigger the immune system to release an antibody to defend the body against infection and disease. When harmless substances like pollen are mistaken for harmful antigens by the immune system, allergy results.

Antihistamine A chemical that counteracts the effects of histamine, a chemical released during allergic reactions.

Antioxidants Substances which inhibit oxidation by destroying free radicals. Common antioxidants are vitamins A, C, E and the minerals selenium and zinc.

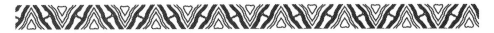

Antiseptic   A preparation which has the ability to destroy undesirable micro-organisms.

Artherosclerosis   A disorder caused when fats are deposited in the lining of the artery wall.

Atopy   A predisposition to various allergic conditions like asthma, hay fever, urticaria and eczema.

Auto-immune disease   A condition in which the immune system attacks the body's own tissue e.g. rheumatoid arthritis.

Autonomic nervous system   Part of the nervous system which controls the involuntary and autonomic function of organs. It consists of a network of nerves divided into two parts: the sympathetic nervous system and the parasympathetic nervous system.

Benign   Non-cancerous cells; not malignant.

Beta carotene   A plant substance which can be converted into vitamin A.

Bile   Liquid produced in the liver for fat digestion.

Candida albicans   Yeast-like fungi found in the mucous membranes of the body.

Carcinogen   Cancer-causing substance or agent.

Cartilage   Connective tissue that forms part of the skeletal system, such as the joints.

Chi   Chinese term for the energy that circulates through the meridians.

Cholesterol   A fat compound, manufactured in the body, that facilitates the transportation of fat in the bloodstream.

Chronic   A disorder that persists for a long time; in contrast to acute.

Cirrhosis   Liver disease caused by damage of the cells and internal scarring *(fibrosis)*.

Collagen   Main component of the connective tissue.

Constitutional treatment   Treatment determined by an assessment of a person's physical, mental and emotional states.

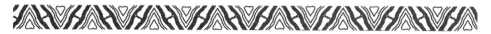

Contagious A term referring to a disease that can be transferred from one person to another by direct contact.

Corticosteroids Drugs used to treat inflammation similar to corticosteroid hormones produced by the adrenal glands that control the body's use of nutrients and excretion of salts and water in urine.

Detoxification Treatment to eliminate or reduce poisonous substances *(toxins)* from the body.

Diuretic Substance that increases urine flow.

DNA A molecule carrying genetic information in most organisms.

Double-blind placebo controlled trials A type of trial to compare the benefits of a treatment where neither the patients nor the doctors know which patients are receiving treatment and which are on a placebo – an inert substance given in place of the drug/ treatment being tested.

Elimination diet A diet which eliminates allergic foods.

Endorphins Substances which have the property of suppressing pain. They are also involved in controlling the body's response to stress.

Enzyme A protein catalyst that speeds chemical reactions in the body.

Essential fatty acids Substances that cannot be made by the body and therefore need to be obtained from the diet.

Free radicals Highly unstable atom or group of atoms containing at least one unpaired electron.

Gene marker Indication of a particular gene defect, in a specific fragment of DNA, determined in laboratory tests.

Hepatic Pertaining to the liver.

Histamine A chemical released during an allergic reaction, responsible for redness and swelling that occur in inflammation.

Holistic medicine Any form of therapy aimed at treating the whole person – mind, body and spirit.

Lymphocyte A type of white blood cell found in lymph nodes. Some lymphocytes are important in the immune system.

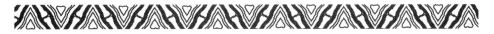

Malignant   A term that describes a condition that gets progressively worse, resulting in death.

Meridians   Energy pathways that connect the acupuncture and acupressure points and the internal organs.

Mucous membrane   Pink tissue that lines most cavities and tubes in the body, such as the mouth, nose etc.

Mucus   The thick fluid secreted by the mucous membranes.

Neurotransmitter   A chemical that transmits nerve impulses between nerve cells.

Oxidation   Chemical process of combining with oxygen or of removing hydrogen.

Parasympathetic nervous system   Also part of the autonomic system, the parasympathetic nervous system is concerned with the body's everyday functions, such as digestion and excretion. It slows down the heart rate and stimulates the organs of the digestive tract.

Placebo   A chemically inactive substance given instead of a drug, often used to compare the efficacy of medicines in clinical trials.

Potency   A term used in homoeopathy to describe the number of times a substance has been diluted.

Prostaglandin   Hormone-like compound manufactured from essential fatty acids.

Sclerosis   Process of hardening or scarring.

Stimulant   A substance that increases energy.

Sympathetic nervous system   Part of the autonomic nervous system, primarily concerned with preparing the body for action in times of stress or excitement. It stimulates functions such as heart rate, sweating and increased blood flow to the body.

Toxin   A poisonous protein produced by disease-causing bacteria.

Vaccine   A preparation given to induce immunity against a specific infectious disease.

Vitamin   Essential nutrient that the body needs to act as a catalyst in normal processes of the body.

Withdrawal   Termination of a habit-forming substance.

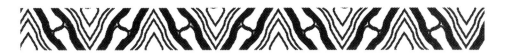

INDEX

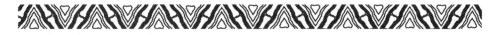

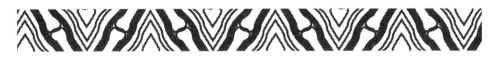

THE NATURAL MEDICINES SOCIETY

The Natural Medicines Society is a registered charity representing the consumer voice for freedom of choice in medicine. The Society needs the support of every individual who uses natural medicines and who is concerned about their continued existence in order to achieve the necessary changes needed to accomplish their wider availability and acceptance within the NHS.

The Society's aims are to improve the standing and practice of natural medicine by encouraging education and research, and by co-operating with the government and the EC on their registration, safety and efficacy. A major drawback in this work has been that none of the Department of Health's licensing bodies has any experts from these systems of medicine sitting on their committees – this has meant that not one of the natural medicines assessed by them has been judged by anyone with an understanding of the therapy's practice. Since the formation of the Society, it has worked towards the establishment of expert representation on the committees appraising these medicines.

To fulfil these aims, the NMS formed the Medicines Advisory Research Committee in February 1988. Known as MARC, its members are doctors, practitioners, pharmacists and other experts in natural medicines. It is the members of MARC who undertake much of the necessary technical and legal work. They have discussed and submitted proposals to the Department of Health's Medicines Control Agency (MCA), on how the EC Directive for Homoeopathic Medicinal Products can be incorporated into the existing UK system, and how medicines outside the orthodox range can be fairly evaluated.

The EC Directive for Homoeopathic Medicinal Products was eventually passed as European law in September 1992, incorporating anthroposophical and biochemic medicines, as well as homoeopathic. With discussions regarding the implementation of

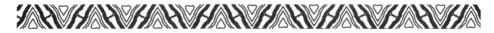

the Homoeopathic Directive now in progress, the MARC's work begins in earnest.

In July 1993, the MCA sent out their consultation paper regarding the implementation of the Directive, which incorporates many of the suggestions submitted by MARC. In it they propose to set up a committee of experts to advise on the registration of homoeopathic, anthroposophic and biochemic medicines. This is a major step forward for the Society, and homoeopathy in general.

With MARC members becoming increasingly involved in the legislative process of the implementation of the Directive, the Natural Medicines Society can now move forward from the short-term aim of protecting the availability of the medicines, to the longer-term aims of promoting and developing their usage and status by instigating and supporting research and education. The NMS has already sponsored some research – it is important to stress here that the Society does not endorse, support or condone animal experimentation – including an expedition to the rain forests in search of medicinal plants, supporting a cancer research project at the Royal London Homoeopathic Hospital and contributing to a methodology Research Fellowship. On the educational side, the Society has published two booklets, with several more planned and has co-sponsored a seminar for doctors and medical students.

The Natural Medicines Society depends upon its membership to continue this unique and important work – please add your support by joining us.

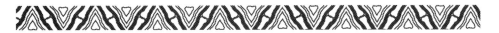

IF YOU ARE NOT ALREADY A MEMBER
WHY NOT JOIN THE
NATURAL MEDICINES SOCIETY?

Mr/Mrs/Miss/Ms _____ (BLOCK CAPITALS PLEASE)

Address _____

_____

Postcode _____ Tel. No. _____

There is no 'fixed' annual membership fee. Please indicate below the amount you wish to pay: minimum £5 (students and unwaged); European countries £15; non-EC £20.

£5 _____ £10 _____ £15 _____

N.B. Pay by Deed of Covenant and/or Direct Debit if you can—please ask for details.

Donations and offers of practical help are also always welcome to aid our fight to return natural medicines to the mainstream of medical practice.

I enclose a donation of £ _____

Please return this form with your remittance (cheques and PO's payable to The Natural Medicines Society), to:

THE NMS MEMBERSHIP OFFICE,
EDITH LEWIS HOUSE,
ILKESTON,
DERBYS,
DE7 8EJ.

(Registered charity no.327468)

You will receive your Membership Card, Member's Handbook, Quarterly Newsletter.

Author Profiles

Hasnain Walji is a writer and freelance journalist specialising in health, nutrition and complementary therapies, with a special interest in dietary supplementation. A contributor to several journals on environmental and Third World consumer issues, he was the founder and editor of *The Vitamin Connection – An International Journal of Nutrition, Health and Fitness*, published in the UK, Canada and Australia, focusing on the link between health and diet. He also launched Healthy Eating, a consumer magazine focusing on the concept of a well-balanced diet, and has written a script for a six-part television series, *The World of Vitamins*, shortly to be produced by a Danish Television company. His latest book, *The Vitamin Guide-Essential Nutrients for Healthy Living*, has just been published, and he is currently involved in developing NutriPlus™: a nutrition database and diet analysis programme for an American software development company.

Dr Andrea Kingston MB ChB, DRCOG, MRCGP, DCH is a Buckinghamshire GP in a five-doctor training practice who has for some years been interested in complementary approaches to healthcare as well as psychiatry and Neuro-linguistic Programming. Hypnotherapy is her major interest, and she has used this technique to help patients throughout the last eight years. As a company doctor to Volkswagen Audi, she contributes regular articles to the company magazine, *Link*. In the past, she has served as a member of the Family Practitioners Committee and as the President of the Milton Keynes Medical Society.

Books by the same authors in the Headway Healthwise series:
- Skin Conditions
- Asthma & Hay Fever
- Headaches & Migraine
- Alcohol, Smoking, Tranquillisers
- Heart Health

Headway

Your Health in Your Hands

HEADWAY LIFEGUIDES

Simple and practical introductions to complementary therapies for the complete beginner.

Tai Chi
0 340 60008 X
£8.99

Alexander Technique
0 340 59680 5
£8.99

Herbalism
0 340 56575 6 £7.99

Aromatherapy
0 340 55950 0 £7.99

Homoeopathy
0 340 56578 0 £7.99

Massage
0 340 55949 7 £7.99

Reflexology
0 340 55594 7 £7.99

Shiatsu
0 340 55321 9 £7.99

Yoga
0 340 55948 9 £7.99

PUBLISHING SEPTEMBER 1994

Visualisation
0 340 61107 3
£6.99

Acupressure
0 340 61106 5
£6.99

HEADWAY HEALTHWISE

Self-help guides to managing common problems using integrated complementary and orthodox approaches. Endorsed by The Natural Medicines Society.

NEW SERIES

Asthma and Hay Fever
0 340 60558 8

Skin Conditions
0 340 60559 6

Alcohol, Smoking, Tranquillisers
0 340 60561 8

Headaches and Migraine
0 340 60560 X

Arthritis and Rheumatism
0 340 60563 4

Heart Health
0 340 60562 6

£6.99 each

Headway is an imprint of
Hodder & Stoughton
A MEMBER OF THE HODDER HEADLINE GROUP